MW01070742

FERTILITY

Healthy Natural Fertility and Pregnancy Guide

DISCOVER NATURAL WAYS TO COMBAT
COMMON FERTILITY PROBLEMS

JOY LOUIS

©**Copyright 2015 Great Reads Publishing, LLC - All rights reserved.**

This document is geared towards providing exact and reliable information in regards to the topic and issue covered. The publication is sold with the idea that the publisher is not required to render accounting, officially permitted, or otherwise, qualified services. If advice is necessary, legal or professional, a practiced individual in the profession should be ordered.

From a Declaration of Principles which was accepted and approved equally by a Committee of the American Bar Association and a Committee of Publishers and Associations.

In no way is it legal to reproduce, duplicate, or transmit any part of this document in either electronic means or in printed format. Recording of this publication is strictly prohibited and any storage of this document is not allowed unless with written permission from the publisher. All rights reserved.

The information provided herein is stated to be truthful and consistent, in that any liability, in terms of inattention or otherwise, by any usage or abuse of any policies, processes, or directions contained within is the solitary and utter responsibility of the recipient reader. Under no circumstances will any legal responsibility or blame be held against the publisher for any reparation, damages, or monetary loss due to the information herein, either directly or indirectly.

The information herein is offered for informational purposes solely, and is universal as so. The presentation of the information is without contract or any type of guarantee assurance.

The trademarks that are used are without any consent, and the publication of the trademark is without permission or backing by the trademark owner. All trademarks and brands within this book are for clarifying purposes only and are the owned by the owners themselves, not affiliated with this document.

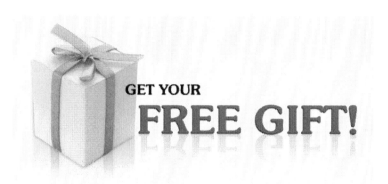

WAIT! – DO YOU LIKE FREE BOOKS?

My **FREE Gift** to You!! As a way to say **Thank You** for downloading my book, I'd like to offer you more **FREE BOOKS!** Each time we release a NEW book, we offer it first to a small number of people as a test–drive. Because of your commitment here in downloading my book, I'd love for you to be a part of this group. You can join easily

here → http://joylouisbooks.com/

Table of Contents

INTRODUCTION 5

CHAPTER ONE   Preparing Your Body for Pregnancy... 9

CHAPTER TWO   Natural Ways to Combat Common

                     Fertility Problems 32

CHAPTER THREE   Common Structural and

                     Anatomical Causes and

                     Solutions for Infertility 88

CHAPTER FOUR   Cupuncture 113

CHAPTER FIVE   Chiropractic Treatments 119

CHAPTER SIX   Pregnancy After 40 123

After Thoughts 127

Glossary of Terms 131

Bibliography 140

Conclusion 147

INTRODUCTION

The dream of many women is to become pregnant, feel the growth of a child inside her, and endure labor pains in order to experience the miracle of childbirth. This is easier said than done for some women. I've seen firsthand the agony and anguish women and men go through when conception seems like an impossibility. I have friends and relatives who have experienced this devastation. Watching their hopes rise and crash each month is heartbreaking. Their doctors did tests, prescribed medications, and performed procedures but to no avail. None of these couples looked into natural ways to conceive, gave up hope, and adopted. Adoption is a beautiful, wonderful, life-saving gift, but it can't replace carrying and delivering your own child. I felt compelled to investigate natural options to solve infertility, and this book is the result of my research and my desire to help those struggling to conceive.

I figured I would have no problem finding a plethora of information on the internet, my local library, and even my closest doctor's office. What I found was: most articles were outdated (written before 2012), much of the information was repetitive, and many unqualified people have fancy looking websites and lots of hot air to spew. I wanted to present as much information on this topic with as much accuracy as possible. Those people struggling to conceive want answers, proven results, and don't want to spend hours, days, weeks to find what they are looking for. My hope is this book will answer your questions about natural fertility methods for women aged twenty to forty-five, explain common male and female fertility problems and solutions, give a structured plan on how to get pregnant, list supplements, exercise, and dietary needs for pre-conception, and discuss the psychological side of getting pregnant.

I also became aware of the insensitivity of many people in the general public and medical field in regards to infertility and the desire to use all-natural methods to aid conception. First, traditional doctors usually want to go the route of medications and procedures to help with fertility. I swear they receive a major kick back from the pharmaceutical companies. They rarely want to discuss natural, holistic ways to approach medical issues. I've heard of doctors actually rolling their eyes at couples requesting natural solutions. I know from personal experience three of my doctors (ob/gyn, G.P., and psychiatrist) always suggest drugs as the first choice of treatment.

Second, if you mention to people you are trying to conceive or are having difficulty getting pregnant, everyone and their brother feel it's appropriate to share their story, whether it relates to you or not. I remember when I was eight months pregnant, every woman I ran into decided to tell me about her nightmarish labor and delivery. Everyone thinks they're an expert because they've been pregnant. Guess what? You're not! Couples who are trying to conceive are usually emotional; they've made the decision to bring another life into this world, and that decision should not be taken lightly. Sharing horror stories and making light of the situation is not comforting. At some baby showers I've attended, the guests are asked to share their best advice with the mommy-to-be. My advice—don't listen to anyone's advice. Every conception, pregnancy, and delivery is unique. Let each woman experience the ups and downs for herself. If she asks for your thoughts, then share. Otherwise wish her well and keep your mouth shut.

Third, I was blessed not to have trouble getting pregnant, but a month or so after my daughter was born, my hormones and emotions went on the ride from hell. I wasn't diagnosed with postpartum depression, but I knew something was wrong. I constantly feared my child's life was in danger, my anger would quickly spiral out of control, and I cried every night because "I was the worst mother." Unfortunately, seventeen years ago natural approaches to my symptoms weren't easily found. I felt trapped and went the route of traditional doctors and medication—lots of medication. I was put on anti-psychotics, anti-depressants, and mood stabilizers. These medications created a situation where I was advised to not get pregnant again. I was told my life and the life of my unborn child would be at serious risk. I didn't know there were options; the internet was too new to be considered reliable and the idea of natural and holistic approaches to my problems was foreign. If a book like this existed seventeen years ago, maybe my daughter wouldn't be an only child.

Bringing a new life into this world is a blessing that can't be truly understood until experienced firsthand. This book is designed to help women conceive naturally, so they can experience the joy and wonder of childbirth.

CHAPTER ONE

PREPARING YOUR BODY FOR PREGNANCY

Controlling what happens inside our bodies seems impossible. Healthy systems and organs operate without our assistance, so we tend to think we shouldn't mess with them. If it ain't broke, don't fix it. But we shouldn't wait until there is a problem to take care of our bodies. Even if you're not thinking about pregnancy, you should still do "preventative maintenance to keep your insides running like new."

We are becoming a nation looking for sustainable food sources, frequenting farmers' markets, and going organic. If you haven't jumped on this bandwagon, hurry up. The Food and Drug Administration (FDA) and the United Stated Department of Agriculture (USDA) allow a certain amount of chemicals into our "fresh" foods. Processed food is laced with toxins and chemicals. We may not immediately feel the effects of these poisons, but they are at work inside us slowly destroying our bodies' systems. Fear not, you can begin to reverse some of the damage you may have done. One way to do this is through a detoxifying diet. Cleansing your body before bringing another life into it is vital. You want the most welcoming, safe environment for your unborn child. Think of this step as baby-proofing your body.

Women planning to conceive need to know that a healthy diet promotes healthy ovulation and helps prevent recurrent miscarriages. Your food intake can affect the body for 90 days after ingestion.

Begin by asking your partner to join you in this detox process. When steps are taken together, you will feel closer to each other, you will both be taking steps to prepare for parenthood, and you will provide support to each other and having support makes all things easier. And many of the foods included in a healthy diet can have a positive effects on your partner's sperm. Guys, your health is just as important as hers! Detoxing isn't as scary as some people think. It is a simple, natural way to cleanse your body of built-up toxins and waste and rid your diet of unwanted sugars, fats, and processed ingredients our bodies aren't meant to consume. Detoxifying is a gradual process, so don't think you have to give up everything at once. Also, those fad diet pills and drinks that say they detox your body quickly don't really work. Remember all things worth doing are worth doing right. The recommended length of time for a detox program varies. I've read that one week of adhering to an all organic, raw foods diet is enough to feel a drastic difference in energy levels. More serious, enthusiastic detoxers aim for a twenty-one day regimen. However long you plan on committing to these dietary changes is up to you but don't stop using what you've learned and return to your old habits after your detox time is up. Hopefully you will make these changes a permanent part of your diet. Beginning a healthy eating routine now will carry over to post-pregnancy eating as well as introducing your child to the healthiest diet possible once he or she begins eating solids.

Step 1

Really look at your current diet. How often do you go to a fast-food restaurant for convenience's sake? Or just because you have a craving? Come on now, be honest. Do you drink soft drinks, diet or regular? How much water do you consume daily? Are you so short on time that dinner comes from a box or the frozen dinner aisle at the supermarket? Consider this—all processed food, those foods with artificial preservatives, meats from animals that received growth hormones and antibiotics, and dairy products that aren't organic—all of these foods are subject to recalls by the government.

I freak out when my car gets recalled for a minor safety issue. But my food?! Yikes. To eliminate the chances of eating tainted foods, go organic!

Step 2

Start by reading the labels on all your foods and drinks. If there is something listed in the ingredients that you can't pronounce, don't put it into your body. Look at the size of the chicken breasts you buy. Are they larger than your Thanksgiving turkey's breast? (I wish mine were as big and firm as some I've seen in grocery stores.) If so, don't buy them. This is a good indication the bird was fed growth hormones. The use of over 440 pesticides are intended to keep crops pest resistant, but these same chemicals then become part of the plant we eat. Growth hormones for animals are causing humans to become resistant to medical antibiotics, plus they change nature's intended growth rate. Look for words like "No GMOs" (Growth Modified Organisms), "grass fed," and "free range." If you purchase 100% organic foods, you will not have to worry about recalls, chemicals, or ingredients you can't pronounce. "What you stop eating can be more important that what you do eat." (*Raw Food page 170*)

Step 3

I understand that buying all organic foods and drinks is expensive. Believe me, I've tried to go completely organic/farm raised, and I couldn't afford it. But you can still make some changes that will help. First, stop buying all processed foods. Homemade food takes more time and effort, but health is more important than time. No more trips to the drive-thru. Period. No more soda of any kind. Stop consuming caffeine in all its forms. (Be prepared for a nasty caffeine-withdrawal headache if you consume three or more cups of coffee a day on a regular basis. These are painful!) Grab a glass of water instead. **You should drink half your body weight in ounces of water each day!** Start eating a more "whole foods" diet—foods that come in their natural state. Some people may go the route of a "raw foods" diet. This diet is defined in the *Raw Food: A Complete Guide to Every Meal of the Day* as "food made from fruits, berries, vegetables, seeds, nuts, dried fruit, algae, sprouts, legumes, honey, cold-pressed oil, and spices. These ingredients are never heated above 104°F." By keeping the foods below the 104° mark, you are retaining more of the nutrients. If you're straddling the fence about trying the raw food approach, maybe this will lean you all the way over the fence—Jinjee Talifero says this about a raw foods diet and pregnancy:

But it was my experience giving birth that convinced me to go 100% raw once and for all! For my first child, I had been eating cooked foods throughout the pregnancy, and the labor was 30 hours—and painful. For my second, I stuck to raw food, and the labor was 2 hours, and almost completely pain free. My third, I was back to cooked food, and it was 40 hours—and painful. That was enough. I wanted another delivery like the short, painless one! For then on, I stuck to raw food and my last two labors were very quick, and relatively pain free.

That's pretty persuasive!

Step 4

Now that you've started with some basics, let's get down to a more serious detox approach. You should begin the day with a glass of lemon water to stimulate the cleansing process. An herbal tea is a good substitute for coffee. And try a smoothie for breakfast. Load your blender with uncooked leafy greens like kale, spinach, arugula, chard, romaine lettuce, etc. (These are absolute must have ingredients!), add a banana or avocado for a creamy texture, core and chop a pear or green apple, add a mixture of frozen berries, and finally add fresh lemon juice from half a lemon. Blend until smooth. This may seem too adventurous for you, but you won't know until you try.

Here are some suggested options:

- Use pure fruit juices instead of the lemon juice.

- Try cucumbers.

- Add chia or flax seed to boost protein and fiber.

- Unsweetened coconut or almond milk adds creaminess and sweetness.

- Add ice before blending to make it a frozen smoothie.

If you truly can't stomach the greens, here is an alternative: unsweetened almond milk, pure, unsweetened pumpkin puree or a peeled, cooked sweet potato, a couple tablespoons of almond butter, one banana, and a sprinkling of cinnamon or pumpkin pie spices.

Snacks are an important part of a healthy diet, so here are some good choices:

- Raw, unsalted pumpkin seeds, almonds, and pistachios.

- Apples and pears dipped in almond butter.

- Uncooked veggies dipped in organic hummus.

- Drink any left-over smoothies.

There are so many good lunch and dinner recipes that it's hard to choose, so I am going to give you a list of ingredients to always have on hand for a healthy meal:

- Grains: quinoa, lentils, black or brown rice, sprouted breads.

- Beans: black, white, and garbanzo (chick peas), navy, pinto.

- Eggs: farm fresh.

- Chicken and turkey: buy only free range or cage free.

- Seafood: mussels, clams, shrimp-must not be canned. Any fresh cold water fish like salmon-farm-raised fish contain dyes and anitboitics. Steer clear of deep water fish like ahi tuna, swordfish, and Chilean sea bass because they may contain mercury.

- Dairy: organic only. Hemp and almond milk are excellent alternatives to cow's milk (There is a school of thought that humans are not meant to consume cow's milk or any products made with cow's milk. I will let you decide this for yourself.)

- Nuts: walnuts and almonds (all in raw form-not roasted and no salt)

- Seeds: flax, hemp, chia, pumpkin, sesame, sunflower (all in raw form with no salt).

- Red meat: must be grass fed! No if, ands, or pork butts! And never undercooked.

- Water: Drink water that has been purified. Reverse osmosis or distilled water is uptimal. Avoid water bottled in plastic-chemicals in plastic can leach into water.

- **Foods to AVOID!!! Soy, semolina, white bread, processed, artificial, and refined sugar, juice that have added sugar, white rice.**

If you do not consider yourself a chef, browse the internet for whole food recipes and detoxifying recipes that include the above ingredients and stay off the television chefs' sites! These lists are in no way complete. They are some basics and will give you a great start to cleansing your body and developing better, healthier eating habits for yourself, your baby, and all your family members.

A healthy diet must include ways to get the needed vitamins, antioxidants, and minerals. Here is a list of some key nutrients, what they do for our bodies, and what foods contain them.

Vitamin D – Creates sex hormones which affect ovulation and hormonal balance

Found in eggs, fatty fish like salmon

Vitamin E – Improves sperm health and motility. (Told you guys!) Deficiency in vitamin E can cause infertility. An antioxidant that protects sperm and egg DNA integrity. Found in raw, unsalted sunflower seeds and almonds, olives, papaya, spinach and other dark leafy greens

Vitamin A – Boosts immune function and is essential for gene transcription.

Found in sweet potatoes, carrots, dark leafy greens, winter squashes, lettuce, dried apricots, cantaloupe, bell peppers, fish, liver, and tropical fruits.

Potassium – Maintains fluid and electrolyte balance which prevents fatigue, irritability, and high blood pressure.

Found in beans, dark leafy greens, potatoes, squashes, yogurt, fish, avocados, mushrooms, and bananas.

Calcium – Necessary for strong bones and teeth, nerve signaling, and secretion of certain hormones and enzymes.

Found in dark leafy greens, organic cheese, milk, and yogurt, bok choy, okra, broccoli, green beans, and almonds.

CoQ10 – Necessary so every cell in the body can produce energy. Improves ova and sperm health. Necessary for sperm motility in semen. Protects cells from free radicals which can damage DNA.

Found in seafood and organ meat

Vitamin C – Improves hormone levels. Increases fertility in women with luteal phase defect. Improves sperm quality, protects sperm DNA, and prevents sperm from clumping.

Found in red bell peppers, broccoli, cranberries, cabbage, potatoes, tomatoes, zucchini, acorn squash, and citrus fruit

Lipoic Acid – Protects female reproductive organs. Improves sperm quality and motility. Helps body reuse antioxidants already in body.

Small amounts found in potatoes, spinach, and red meat

B6 – Regulates hormones and blood sugar. Alleviates PMS symptoms. May ease morning sickness. Helps with Luteal Phase Defect.

Found in tuna, bananas, turkey, liver, salmon, cod, spinach, bell peppers, turnip, mustard, and collard greens, garlic, cauliflower, celery, cabbage, asparagus, broccoli, kale, Brussels sprouts, chard

B12–Improves sperm quality and production. Boosts endometrium which can lower risks of miscarriages.

Found in clams, oysters, mussels, liver, caviar, lobster, beef, lamb, cheese, and eggs.

Folic acid – Helps prevent neural tube defects, congenital heart defects, cleft lips, limb defects, and urinary tract anomalies in the developing fetus.

Found in liver, lentils, pinto black, navy, kidney, and garbanzo beans, asparagus, spinach, collard greens

Selenium – Protects egg and sperm from free radical which can cause chromosomal damage which in turn can cause miscarriages and birth defects. Necessary for sperm production.

Found in liver, snapper, cod, halibut, tuna, salmon, sardines, shrimp, crimini mushrooms, turkey, and Brazil nuts. **Zinc** – Works in conjunction with over 300 other enzymes to keep body functioning properly. Needed for cell division. Maintains estrogen and progesterone balance which ensures reproductive system operating at optimal performance. Low levels of zinc in early pregnancy linked to miscarriages. For men, increasing zinc will boost sperm levels, form, and function. Decreases male infertility.

Found in calf liver, oysters, beef lamb, venison, sesame seeds, pumpkin seeds, yogurt, turkey, green peas, shrimp.

Iron – Low levels can cause anovulation (lack of ovulation) and poor egg health.

Found in lentils, spinach, sesame and pumpkin seeds, kidney, garbanzo, and navy beans, venison, molasses, acorn squash, and beef.

Essential Fatty Acids – Regulates hormones, increases cervical mucus, promotes ovulation, improves uterine health. Contain DHA and EPA. Low EPA may cause premature birth, low birth weight, and hyperactivity.

Found in flax seeds walnuts, salmon, sardines, halibut, shrimp, snapper, scallops, chia seeds.

Fats – Essential to development of fetus.

Found in coconut oil, grass-fed meats, fish, nuts, and seeds.

Proteins – Include animal and vegetable sources of protein daily.

Found in grass-fed beef and pork, free-range/cage-free turkey and chicken, farm-fresh eggs, wild caught catfish, Pollack, salmon, tilapia, clams, and shrimp.

Fiber – Gets rid of excess estrogen and xenohormones.

Found in acorn squash, corn, white, black, kidney, and garbanzo beans, avocados, whole wheat bread and pasta, brown rice, lentils, pears (with skin), artichokes, raspberries, peas, broccoli, apples (with skin), almonds, and barley.

Another vital aspect of preparing your body for pregnancy is exercise. This is also something you and your partner can do together. And just like the changes in diet, hopefully these changes in exercise will be ongoing. Pregnancy is exhausting and exercise and movement can help you regain some of that lost energy. During my first trimester, I was exhausted at 4:00 every afternoon, just like clockwork. This was a huge problem; I was driving home from work at 4:00. After almost falling asleep behind the wheel, I had to change my afternoon schedule. Thankfully, my job provided some flexibility, and I was able to leave a half hour earlier so I could be home before the 4:00 witching hour. I started walking at least a mile a day—fall, winter, and spring—unless the sidewalks were icy. My energy returned as well as a happier demeanor.

There are so many activities to choose from, but picking one that you can continue during pregnancy is something to consider. Also choose an activity that you are willing to do for at least 30 minutes five or more days a week. Walking, yoga, and swimming are three great options. Look into your local health clubs, park district gyms and facilities, and community exercise classes if you feel you need the help of other people to stay motivated and on track. Also, doing classes with other pregnant women will allow you to meet new, supportive, understanding women. Those of you who have good self-discipline can look online for yoga or pregnancy workout videos. Of course, check with your doctor before beginning any exercise routine. Make sure to stay hydrated, stop before exhausted, avoid activities on uneven surfaces so as not to fall, wear a heavy-duty support bra, and listen to your body. Your body will change with each trimester and your exercise routine may need to be altered as well.

Yoga is a fantastic way to stay limber, tone muscles, improve balance and circulation, all without impact on your joints. Yoga also teaches deep breathing to relieve stress, relax your entire body, refocus, and cleanse toxins from your body. These breathing techniques will be very useful during natural child birth. They also help keep blood pressure low, even in painful and stressful situations. It's not about sitting cross-legged, thumb and forefinger touching, and repeating, "Om." This is definitely an exercise you will need to alter once you are pregnant. Certain stretches and poses are not recommended during pregnancy. But properly practicing yoga during pregnancy will help offset the demands pregnancy make on your body. It will also keep you connected and more present during this amazing experience. Yoga increases your flexibility, strengthens your body, and calms your mind. As you twist your body, you are detoxifying your body. The twists not only feel good, but they are putting pressure on internal organs so they can eliminate waste and toxins. Many of us carry our stress in our necks, shoulders, lower back, and hips. These areas can also be affected by our posture and daily activities. Yoga will work all those areas of the body each time we practice it. We will also be releasing emotional stress that we may not even realize we are holding on to.

I practice yoga on an irregular basis, but when I do my body feels aligned and stretched. My tense muscles are relieved. It's almost like going for a chiropractic adjustment. My husband carries all his stress in his shoulders and up the back of his neck. He gets intense stress headaches that are so painful he has to go to sleep to ease the pain. He will sometimes wake up the next morning and still have the same headache. He has gone to a chiropractor in the past and gotten great relief, but our bank account couldn't handle what the insurance wouldn't cover. I keep telling him he should give yoga a try. His response is always the same, "I don't bend that way." Well, dear, very few people do bend that way at first. You just need to work at your own pace and allow your body to slowly loosen and become more flexible.

Walking is a fabulous exercise during pregnancy because you can do it through all trimesters and your partner can do it with you. Make sure you have supportive shoes that are meant for walking, not jogging or running; the supports are different depending on the activity. Unlike during some exercises, you can carry on a conversation. This is a great opportunity for the parents-to-be to discuss their hopes, fears, and dreams of parenting. It's a good time to clear the air if things are bothering you.

Swimming is virtually impact free and will lighten your load so to speak. Short of traveling beyond the atmosphere, swimming provides that closest thing to weightlessness. Believe me, when you feel like you're carrying the weight of a fetal elephant, being able to ease the burden of that extra weight feels fantastic. The benefits of swimming include a cardiovascular workout, improved circulation, and increased tone and strength in the large muscles like your arms and legs. A morning swim might even counteract morning sickness.

Getting your body in physical condition before pregnancy and maintaining an exercise regimen during pregnancy help strengthen muscles that will be used in labor and core muscles which are needed to help support your back. It will help you get your figure back after delivery. Plus it provides a healthy, strong environment in which your baby can grow.

A third and extremely important aspect of your health is to prepare emotionally and mentally for this life-changing event. An entire book could be written on the emotional roller coaster that pregnancy sends women on. In this book, I decided to address some of the emotional stressors while trying to get pregnant. Before you buy a car, you research what make and model you like, find out its gas mileage, compare prices, and take test drives. Before you buy a house or rent an apartment, you research the neighborhood, look at multiple options, and figure out just how much you can afford to spend each month. Even before you vote you do research. So why would you spend less time discussing an even more important life decision?

Your mental and psychological health can create stress and anxiety during pregnancy which can affect your developing baby. Depression and anxiety and mood disorders before, during, and after pregnancy are common mental and emotional health concerns. Using prescription drugs to combat these issues put you and your unborn child at risk. According to the Stanford School of Medicine, the risks to the fetus include teratogenesis, neonatal toxicity, and long-term neurobehavioral effects. Teratogenesis is the development of congenital malformations such as cleft lip or palate and affects the development of the fetal organs and organ systems. During the prenatal stages, toxicity can directly affect the fetus' central nervous system. The effects of this exposure will be most noticeable in physical and behavioral symptoms shown in the first month after birth. I personally know the damaging effects of psychiatric medications on my body after pregnancy. I was told my mental health was so dependent on strong prescription medications, that I would never be able to go off them long enough to have a safe pregnancy. One medication is tied to such horrific birth defects, I had to sign a waiver stating I would not get pregnant while taking this medication and if I did, I was fully aware of the risks to my unborn child. That scared me so much, my husband and I agreed to take all precautions necessary to prevent another pregnancy. If I would have known about the natural ways to ease the symptoms of the mental and emotional conditions I suffer from, I know I would have opted for the natural treatment so we could have other children. Thankfully, you have the information I did not have.

So how can you deal with these issues safely and naturally? Reread the section on diet! There are many foods that help balance hormones, whether you are pregnant or not. Look into these first! In the next chapter, herbs that can help will be discussed. There are options. Choose wisely young grasshopper.

As hard as it can be to wait until both partners feel ready to be parents, it is for the best. Pregnancy is not something to force on someone. I was ready to start a family immediately after our wedding, but my husband wasn't ready. Three years later he felt he was ready to shoulder the responsibilities of fatherhood. It was extremely hard for me to wait, but those three years allowed him to mature which made him a wonderful father. Pregnancy should not be considered a solution for relationship problems. Work out your problems before bringing another person into an unstable situation.

Getting pregnant will alter your life forever. The pregnancy itself starts the change. There are many things you will have to sacrifice during the pregnancy. Are you sure you're prepared mentally and emotionally to face these changes? Here are just a few things to consider:

No caffeine in any form.

- The possibility of frequent vomiting due to morning sickness. Or you may just feel nauseated for long periods. (I spent my first trimester feeling like I had the worst and longest hangover ever.)

- At times you will be exhausted and fall asleep quickly. Other times, you will be exhausted but unable to sleep.

- You will reach a stage when you can't get comfortable in bed, especially if you're a stomach sleeper.

- Some women have the difficult task of not smoking or drinking.

- These issues may seem ridiculous to even mention, but they will affect your emotional and mental health, especially the lack of sleep. Are you ready to face these possibilities on a regular basis? Is your partner ready to support you when you cry easily, get cranky, toss and turn all night trying to get comfortable, and feel like you are as big as a whale? You and your partner will need ways to combat the stresses of pregnancy and trying to get pregnant. Here are some simple suggestions:

- Each of you should set aside time once month to spend with friends. A good laugh is something we all benefit from. However, ladies, you may want to set some ground rules with your friends who are already mothers. First, no talking about the baby, diaper changes, breast feeding, etc. Second, no showing adorable pictures and videos of said child. Seeing how happy other women are because they have what you are struggling to get will lead to a depressing experience. True friends will understand the fragile emotional and mental state you are in and should be more than happy to oblige your ground rules.

- Give each other massages, or find a masseuse who caters to pregnant woman. (There are special tables with a hole for your stomach to rest in.) Some spas will put you both in the same room for a sense of connection. Just make certain that the oils being used are all natural. What we absorb through our skin can affect our internal organs and their systems.

• Enjoy your sexual relationship! Once a baby enters your life, the chances of you both having the energy and desire for sex at the same time will be few and far between. Plus just finding the time to be alone is difficult.

• Here are some suggestions just for the mommy-to-be:

• Read a book that has nothing to do with pregnancy. I remember trying to read as many books as possible on pregnancy and what I was going to experience each step of the way. I found so many books contradicted each other that I became frustrated and angry. Except for the books I borrowed, I threw every one away. I was an emotional mess and just wanted clear answers. Thank goodness the internet wasn't invented. I probably would have pulled my hair out after reading all the information available online.

• Take a relaxing, quiet bath using only natural products. Allow yourself to thoroughly enjoy this luxury. The only baths you will probably experience for the first few years after your baby is born are ones with you on the outside of the tub, bubble bath being splashed all over the bathroom, and toys that you will have to learn to shower around.

- Take naps whenever you can. I cannot stress this one enough. Sleep will become a treasured and horded commodity after the baby is born. When we sleep our bodies recuperate from daily stresses and work to keep us healthy. Sleep is a necessary part of a healthy lifestyle. It is just as important as the food and water we drink. (Funny story, I have a genetic bone growth under my tongue called tori mandibulares. Essentially, I have excessive bone growth along the sides of my jaw bone under my tongue. OK, no big deal. I clench my teeth when stressed, and this action increases and promotes this bone growth. Over the years, the growth has gotten so large that the two sides of my jaw bone almost touch. My point—stress can do all sorts of things to our bodies besides raise blood pressure.)

Once you and your partner are on the same page, have considered all the changes, and are willing to support each other through the ups and downs of the pregnancy and parenthood, then go for it!

CHAPTER TWO

NATURAL WAYS TO COMBAT COMMON FERTILITY PROBLEMS

You and your partner have made the decision to become pregnant. You've altered your diet and started an exercise program you can stick to. But even these great intentions are not allowing you to conceive. What 's the problem? Who can I turn to? Where do I look to find answers? Hopefully, you will choose to tackle these problems using natural methods first. Don't be like me and head straight to the pharmacy, or even more drastic measures—surgical procedures. Conception is natural, so look for natural solutions. And before you jump to infertility conclusions, you must have been trying to conceive for at least one year before you can be considered infertile. Sometimes we see friends and family getting pregnant so quickly it makes your head spin. You start to feel pressure and stress to hurry your process along to keep up with the Joneses. Well, you're not the Joneses so take a step back and breathe.

According to conceiveeasy.com, these are the first things to try:

- Chart and track your cycles, chart and track your cycles, chart and track your cycles. No, the repetition isn't a misprint. Your menstrual cycle can be affected by various outside sources each month and they can create almost unnoticeable changes to drastic ones. Stress is one of the biggest culprits. Understanding your cycle will aid in knowing your most fertile time each month. Fertilization can only occur during ovulation, but just because you are ovulating does not mean you are fertile. The cervical mucus that is discharged changes throughout your cycle. The first few days after the menstrual cycle ends will be dry. As the days pass, the mucus will increase until the peak of ovulation when the mucus is clear slippery and the consistency like that of egg whites.

- Your basal body temperature will also change with the onset of ovulation. Your temperature will be higher. Purchasing a basal thermometer may be wise investment. There are also ovulation predictor kits for purchase that detect the Luteinizing Hormone (LH) in your urine. The LH increases 24 to 48 hours before the start of ovulation. Even women with irregular periods can track their cycles and be successful in recognizing their most fertile time of month. Each woman's cycle is unique. One woman's cycle can be unique from month to month. It is important that you pay attention to your body during this time and not listen to the know-it-alls who have already conceived. We know no two humans are alike, so why should we assume two bodies to be the same?

- In my teens and twenties, anytime I felt stress I would have two periods in one 28-day cycle. In my late twenties through to my late thirties, my period was like clockwork. I could tell the day and time of day my period would begin. So for about ten years I knew what to expect each month. Then my forties hit and I was averaging a period every 18 days. It was also at this time that I was experiencing some of the worst stress of my life. Coincidence? I don't think so.

- Check your diet. The previous chapter's discussion on the importance of certain foods to provide vitamins, nutrients, and minerals can be key to healthy female and male reproduction systems. Don't discount the importance of what you put into your body and the immense impact food and drink have on all of your body's systems and organs.

- Start incorporating fertility herbs into your daily routine. Such herbs can be found in health food stores in their most natural and potent states. (A more complete list of herbs and their benefits will be in the next section.)

- Reduce your stress and the stress of your partner. Men can be just as frustrated as women when conception does not happen quickly. My husband panicked after our first month of trying didn't work. He wanted to change underwear style and make an appointment with the doctor to make sure his "swimmers" were showing up for the big event and were strong enough to complete a lap or two. I had to "stroke" his ego and tell him time was all we needed for now. And three months later I conceived.

The following is only a sampling of the most common herbs used to treat certain fertility problems. The list is constantly changing as new herbs are added. These herbs can be found at health food stores and even grown at home. I am not a doctor nor do I play one on TV; therefore, my research is superficial at best. As with any treatment, consult with your doctor, midwife, or an herbalist before using the herbs and research the dosages appropriate for your age and weight. **There are precautions that accompany each herb, so please read carefully! Almost every herb should NOT be taken once pregnant!**

Herbs to Treat Amenorrhea (Absent period, lack of menstruation)

Having a regular menstruation cycle is vital to knowing when you are at optimal times to conceive. This helps with the tracking and charting necessary each month. Regularity applies to reproduction and not just digestion. Many of these herbs also help develop a stronger, toner uterus. Just imagine, toning and strengthening without going to the gym. Now if I could only do that with the rest of my body.

Dong Quai

- Strengthens uterus, regulates hormones, and improves timing of menstrual cycle. Improves blood circulation to the reproductive system.

- Used to combat stagnation like Polycystic Ovarian Syndrome (PCOS), endometriosis, ovarian cysts, and fibroids.

- Do not continue use once pregnant!

Black Cohosh

- Tones, strengthens, and regulates shedding of uterus.

- Used to regulate the menstrual cycle so tracking and charting ovulation becomes easier.

- Do not continue use once pregnant!

Maca

- Promotes hormone balance, fertility, and sexual virility and nourishes endocrine system.

- Used by women to balance estrogen and progesterone levels which are critical for conception and a healthy pregnancy. Men who take maca may have increased libido, sperm count, and overall healthier reproductive system.

- May cause changes to menstrual cycle when first used. Do not continue using once pregnant.

Motherwart

- Reduces uterine spasms and cramping, improves uterine tone, and mildly stimulate the uterus to bring on menstruation. Excellent for calming anxiety and reducing stress related to trying to conceive.

- Used to treat amenorrhea (absence of menses), dysmenorrhea (painful periods), depression, anxiety, stress, uterine fibroids, ovarian cysts, endometriosis, and Premenstrual Syndrome (PMS).

- Do not continue using once pregnant.

Mogwart

- Encourages menstruation, relieves tension and stress, and aids in absorption of vitamins and minerals.

- Used to treat amenorrhea.

- Do not continue using once pregnant.

Parsley

- Brings on menstruation.

- May continue to use in foods once pregnant. Do not take concentrated does of it once pregnant.

Vitex

- Balances fertility hormones by regulating pituitary gland functions, promotes ovulation, and improves timing of menstrual cycle.

- Used to increase progesterone, lengthen luteal phase, treat mild endometriosis, relieve PMS, regulate menstrual cycle, reduce uterine cysts, stabilize menstruation after stopping birth control pill, stimulates milk production in new mothers.

- Can be taken until the end of the first trimester.

Shatavari

- Promotes regular menstruation by aiding regulation of estrogen levels.

- Used to combat adaptogenic actions (stress), autoimmune fertility issues, support mucus membranes, subside uterine contractions, regulate cycle, increase milk production, and reduce fluid retention.

- Should be used by men and women. Check with doctor, mid-wife, or herbalist if it can be taken during pregnancy.

Tribulus

- Normalizes ovulation, increases serum follicle stimulating hormone (FSH) and estradiol in women, and increases sex hormones in both men and women.

- Used by men to increase testosterone, improve sexual desire, increase count, motility, and health of sperm, produce dehydroepiandrosterone (DHEA) for erectile dysfunction.

- Used by women to improve sexual desire and decrease effects of antisperm antibodies.

- Do not continue using once pregnant.

White Peony

- Builds blood, increases circulation to reproductive organs, balances hormones, encourages menstruation, and promotes relaxation.

- Used to combat dysmenorrhea (painful menstruation) and uterine stagnation conditions (Uterine fibroids, endometriosis, and PCOS).

- Do not continue using once pregnant.

Yarrow

- Stimulates uterus to shed endometrium and stimulates regular menstruation.

- Used to combat painful menstruation, heavy menstruation, and pelvic congestion.

- Do not continue using once pregnant.

Herbs to support healthy cervical mucus (necessary for sperm to reach egg)

Borage Seed Oil

- Increases cervical mucus and balances hormones, reduces stress and PMS symptoms.

- Do not continue using once pregnant or breast-feeding.

Dandelion

- Stimulates mucus membrane secretions and balances hormones.

- Do not continue using once pregnant.

Evening Primrose Oil

- Increases cervical mucus and balances hormones.

- Used to combat symptoms of PMS, increase cervical mucus, tone uterine muscles to prepare for pregnancy.

- Do not continue using once pregnant.

Licorice Root

- Supports endocrine health and promotes mucus membrane secretions.

- Used to combat immunological, stress-related, and inflammatory fertility problems and treat dysmenorrhea.

- Licorice does not interact well with some medications. Please seek advice from a medical or herbal specialist.

Marshmallow Root

- Supports natural functions of mucus membranes.

- Used to soothe and relieve inflammation of mucus membranes.

- Not enough studies have been done on its effects during pregnancy. Consult a medical or herbal specialist.

Oregon Grape Root

- Encourages mucus membranes to secrete and supports liver function which aids hormone balance.

- Do not continue using once pregnant.

Red Clover

- Increases cervical mucus and circulation to the male and female reproductive organs.

- Used to combat vaginal dryness, menstrual cramps, hormone balance, and blocked fallopian tubes.

- Do not use if you have one or more of the following conditions: uterine hyperplasia, endometriosis, uterine fibroids, or any estrogen-sensitive conditions.

Shatavari

- Increases mucus production and acts as anti-inflammatory and reduces adhesions in the entire body.

- Used to reduce stress, combat immune related fertility issues, support mucus membranes, regulate menstrual cycle, and reduces fluid retention.

- Do not continue use once pregnant.

Yarrow

- Tones and moistens mucus membranes.

- Used to combat painful, heavy menstruation, eliminate pelvic congestion, and stimulate menstruation.

- Do not continue using once pregnant.

Herbs to treat endometriosis

Ashwagandha

- Supports overall endocrine system functions.

- Used to encourage proper immune responses and aid in some autoimmune fertility issues.

- Consult herbalist or medical doctor if safe to continue once pregnant.

Bee Propolis

- Extreme anti-inflammatory.

- Used to combat uterine fibroids, endometriosis, ovarian cysts, blocked fallopian tubes, Pelvic Inflammatory Disease (PID), and reproductive trauma or surgeries. Also used to treat recurrent miscarriage, Premature Ovarian Failure, and antisperm antibodies.

- Do not continue using during pregnancy of anyone in either partner's family is allergic to honey or bee stings.

Burdock Root

- Supports liver function which balances hormones.

- Used to combat congested organs and tissues.

- Do not continue using once pregnant.

Castor Oil

- Increases circulation, promotes healing of tissues and organs underneath the skin's surface.

- Used to dissolve foreign tissue growth, stimulate detoxification in liver and lymphatic system, and may prevent disease in reproductive system.

- Do not continue using once ovulation has begun.

Cinnamon Bark

- Reduces heavy menstrual flow and increases circulation to reproductive system to heal congested tissues.

- Used to combat PCOS in women with insulin resistance and reduce endometriosis, unterine fibroids, and menorrhagia.

- Do not continue using once pregnant. Can still use as a spice in food.

Dong Quai

- Increases circulation in order to allow blood to remove excess tissue growth, heal tissue damage, limit scar tissue, and adhesion formation.

- Used to remove toxins, dead tissue, diseased tissue, and metabolic waste. Stimulates healthy immune response and reduces depression, fatigue, and psycho-emotional symptoms in women with endometriosis.

Echinacea

- Supports proper immune function.

- Used to calm flare-ups in the immune system.

- Check with doctor or herbalist to see if you should continue using once pregnant.

Feverfew

- Reduces pain and migraines associated with menstrual cycle.

- Do not continue using once pregnant.

Ginger Root

- Increases circulation and supports digestion.

- Used to combat inflammatory issues.

- Consult doctor or herbalist if can continue use after pregnant.

Goldenseal Root

- Helps prevent scar tissue and adhesion formation.

- Used as an anti-inflammatory.

- Do not continue using once pregnant.

Horsetail Aerial Parts

- Promotes proper tissue growth and bleeding.

- Used as astringent to tone and heal excess foreign tissue.

- Do not continue using once pregnant.

Jamaican Dogwood Root

- Reduces muscular pain associated with foreign tissue growth and bleeding.

- Used as antispasmodic and analgesic.

- Do not continue using once pregnant.

Maca

Helps balance hormones, promotes fertility and sexual virility, and helps defend the body against disease.

- Used to nourish and balance endocrine system and support normal sexual function.

- Do not continue using once pregnant.

Nettles

- Supports healthy iron levels.

- Used to combat excessive menstrual bleeding and promote healthy liver function.

- Consult doctor or herbalist if you can continue using once pregnant.

Red Raspberry Leaf

- Tones uterine muscles, strengthens uterus, boosts egg quality, and normalizes menstrual bleeding.

- Used to contract and shrink internal and external body tissues in order to prevent hemorrhaging.

- Do not continue using once pregnant.

Rehmannia Root

- Reduces inflammation and uterine spasms.

- Used to regulate menstrual cycle, reduce irritability in uterus, and support kidney, heart, and liver health.

- Do not continue using once pregnant.

White Peony

- Increases progesterone levels, lowers testosterone levels, and balances estrogen.

- Used to alleviate pain, encourage relaxation, and circulate blood in pelvic area.

- Do not continue using once pregnant.

Yarrow

- Promotes circulation, reduces excessive bleeding, and relieves pelvic congestion.

- Used to combat uterine fibroids, PCOS, and spasms.

- Do not continue using once pregnant.

Herbs to promote estrogen balance (need liver supporting herbs to naturally detox body of xenoestrogens)

Burdock Root

- Nourishes and cleanses liver.

- Used to remove excess estrogen.

- Do not continue using once pregnant.

Dandelion Root

- Aids in liver health.

- Used to stimulate digestion.

- Do not continue using once pregnant.

Evening Primrose Oil

- Contains Linoleic Acid (LA)—creates prostaglandin E—and Gamma Linolenic Acid (GLA)—synthesizes prostaglandin E.

- Used to regulate hormones, lessen PMS symptoms, increase cervical mucus.

- Do not continue using once pregnant.

Flax Seed

- Contains fiber and lignans (second strongest group of phytoestrogens).

- Used to remove excess estrogen and protect from xenoestrogens.

- Do not continue using once pregnant.

Licorice

- Mimics estrogen.

- Used to support endocrine system by blocking xenohormones from binding.

- Consult herbalist or doctor before continuing use once pregnant.

Maca

- Balances estrogen and progesterone.

- Used as adaptogen, endocrine system tonic, and sexual function normalizer.

Milk Thistle

- Promotes liver health.

- Used to balance hormones and remove excess toxins form body.

- Do not continue using once pregnant.

Red Clover

- Aids in detoxification prior to pregnancy.

- Used to protect body from xenohormones.

- Do not continue using once pregnant.

Seaweed

- Improves estrogen metabolism.

- Used to protect thyroid and strengthen liver, kidneys, bladder, and adrenal glands.

- Consult with doctor or herbalist to find which types of seaweed are safe to consume in small amounts during pregnancy.

Sesame Seed

- Contains six essential fatty acids (EFA) and high amounts of omega 3.

- Used to support estrogen levels and balance hormones.

- Consult doctor or herbalist to learn if consuming sesame seeds during pregnancy is safe.

Shatavari

- Regulates estrogen.

- Used to regulate menstrual cycle.

- Do not continue using once pregnant.

Tribulus

- Vital to male and female fertility.

- Used to normalize ovulation, increase sex hormone production in men and women, improve sexual drive in men and women, increase sperm count, motility, and health, decrease effects of antisperm antibodies, and may help erectile dysfunction (ED).

- Do not continue using once pregnant.

Herbs to treat heavy menstrual bleeding (menorrhagia)

The following herbs are all used to relieve heavy menstrual bleeding. As with all the herbs mentioned so far, do not continue use once pregnant. If you want more unless it is a spice used in food.

Cranesbill

- Used to stop heavy menstrual bleeding or uterine hemorrhaging

Cinnamon

- Curbs heavy menstrual bleeding due to endometriosis and uterine fibroids.

- Can aid with insulin resistance in women with PCOS

Ginger

- Acts as an anti-inflammatory, cleanser, and pain reliever.

- Improves circulation to reproductive organs.

Hibiscus

- High in vitamin C which aids in absorption of iron.

- Normalizes blood pressure. (Notice this says blood pressure, not high or low blood pressure. We hear so much about high blood pressure and its health effects, but low blood pressure is also a concern. I normally have a healthy, low blood pressure, which is amazing considering how easily I stress over simple things. But I was at the doctor's office for a physical and the nurse had to take my BP twice and in different arms. My numbers were so low she asked if I wanted to lie down; she said I shouldn't be walking around with BP this low. I felt fine, and the doctor gave me a clean bill of health. It's never been that low again, but I know from the look on the nurse's face that she was either concerned or thought I was a zombie.)

Liferoot

- Normalizes menstrual cycle.

Maca

- Provides hormone balance.

Nettles

- An astringent.

- High in iron and vitamin C.

Periwinkle

- Curbs mid-cycle spotting/bleeding

Seaweed

- Improves hormone balance.

- High in fiber and iron.

Shepherd's Purse

- Reduces acute heavy bleeding and postpartum hemorrhaging.

Vitex

- Supports hormonal balance and normalizes whole reproductive system.

White Peony

- Increases blood flow to pelvic region.

- Good for uterine stagnation issues.

Yarrow

- Promotes circulation, detoxification, acts as astringent, and strengthens and tightens tissues.

Yellow Dock

- Aids in removal of toxins and supports liver function with high amounts of iron.

Herbs that combat immune related fertility issues. (Body attacks and kills foreign cells associated with reproductive function.)

Ashwagandha

- Supports proper immune responses.

Bee Propolis

- Specifically helps with recurrent miscarriage, Premature Ovarian Failure, and antisperm antibody.

Cordyceps

- Restores human macrophage (type of white blood cell that ingests foreign material) and natural killer cell activities.

Dong Quai

- Stimulates healthy immune responses, healthy mind function, and counteracts inflammation.

Echinacea

- Perfect for use when immune function support is needed immediately.

Licorice

- Supports overall endocrine function.

Maca

- Nourishes pituitary, adrenal, and thyroid glands.

Rehmannia or Di Huang

- Regulates blood pressure and insulin levels and acts as an anti-inflammatory.

Reishi Mushroom

- Down-regulates excessive immune response but enhances monocyte (white blood cells used to regulate immunity), macrophage, and T lymphocyte (cells used to find abnormalities and infections in cells) activity.

Shatavari

- Supports overall immune health.

Shiitake Mushroom

- Stimulates and supports immune system.

Tribulus

- Decreases effects of antisperm antibodies.

Libido Boosting Herbs

The following herbs increase sexual desire and increase circulation to reproductive for men and women. Consult a doctor or herbalist to if you should continue use once pregnant.

Damiana

- Female aphrodisiac, increases circulation, and heightens sexual pleasure.

Epimedium

- Increases male virility and enhances erections in length and hardness.

Maca

- Increases sexual desire in men and women.

- Increases vaginal secretions and increases testosterone in men.

Muira Puama

- Supports healthy erections, male fertility, and increases male libido.

Saffron

- Increases sexual drive and feelings in men and women.

Tribulus

- Overall fertility tonic for women and men.

- Men can experience larger, harder erections which in turn means women can experience that as well!

Vitex

- All-around female reproductive enhancer—boosts libido and enhances sexual pleasure.

Yohimbe

- Supports healthy circulation to reproductive organs, sustains firmer erections, and boosts libido.

Herbs to possibly prevent miscarriages

These herbs are to be used for at least 3 months prior to conception. If you feel you are experiencing a miscarriage, contact your doctor or midwife IMMEDIATELY! Do not administer these herbs as a way to stop a possible miscarriage in progress. Do not use once pregnant.

Black Haw

- Reduces uterine contractions and spasms.

Cramp Bark

- Reduces uterine contractions and uterine muscle spasms.

False Unicorn

- Strengthens uterus and cervix.

Partridge Berry

- Strengthens uterus.

Vitex

- Increases progesterone to avoid recurrent miscarriages.

Wild Yam

- Relieves an irritable uterus.

Herbs to combat ovarian cysts

Ovarian cysts are a result of a failed or disordered ovulation. These herbs will promote hormonal balance, regulate ovulation, improve circulation, and detoxify liver. Do not continue using once pregnant.

Black Cohosh

- Regulates entire menstrual cycle.

Blue Cohosh

- Ovarian and uterine tonic to regulate cycle.

Castor Oil

- Enhances circulation, promotes healing and detoxification of tissues under the skin.

Dong Quai

- Balances hormones, treats congestive fertility problems, and improves circulation to reproductive organs.

Maca

- Helps balance hormones so menstrual cycle can be regular.

Milk Thistle

- Supports liver health which eliminates toxins.

Seaweed

- Improves estrogen metabolism.

Tribulus

- Normalizes ovulation.

Vitex

- Balances hormones, promotes ovulation, and improves timing of menstrual cycle.

- **Wild Yam**

- Promotes healthy cycle.

Yarrow

- Relieves pelvic congestion and improves menstrual timing.

Herbs to combat dysmenorrhea (painful menstruation)

Be sure to ask a doctor, midwife, or herbalist if the pain you are experiencing is truly due to your cycle and not a symptom of a more serious fertility problem. Keep a journal of the timing of the pain in relation to your cycle and specifically where the pain is felt.

Black Cohosh

- Reduces spasms of skeletal muscles associated with pain in lower back and down the thighs.

Black Haw

- Reduces painful cramping.

Chamomile

- Acts as a mild sedative.

Cramp Bark

- Treats exactly what its name states!

Dong Quai

- Pain reducer and anti-inflammatory properties.

Feverfew

- Handles pelvic pain as well as migraines associated with menses.

Ginger

- Soothes upset stomach caused by severe cramping.

Jamaican Dogwood

- Combats even debilitating pain.

Motherwort

- Brings quick relief to painful symptoms.

Red Clover

- Reduces cramping.

Wild Yam

- Reduces muscle spasms in uterus, fallopian tubes, and ovaries.

Herbs to combat PCOS (polycystic ovarian syndrome)

These herbs help balance blood sugar levels, maintain hormone balance, promote healthy digestion and regulate menses and ovulation. Do not continue using once pregnant.

Ashwagandha

- Supports overall endocrine health.

Cinnamon

- Greatly reduces insulin resistance in women.

Burdock

- Helps balance blood sugar levels.

- Cleanses congested tissues and organs.

Eleuthero

- Supports overall endocrine health.

Gymnema

- Destroys sugar.

Licorice

- Balances hormones.

Maca

- Increase progesterone levels in men and women. For women it helps balance estrogen and progesterone levels.

Tribulus

- Reduce ovarian cysts in women with PCOS

Saw Palmetto

- Combats Hirsutism (excessive body hair and thinning of hair on head) of women with PCOS.

Vitex

- Helps regulate cycle.

White Peony

- Lowers serum and free testosterone levels in women with PCOS.

- Better blood circulation in pelvic region.

Herbs to combat poor egg health

These herbs will help relieve stress, balance hormones, improve circulation to reproductive organs, and provide proper endocrine function. These herbs should not be used once pregnant. Are you sick of reading about the same herbs over and over? They provide such important and varied functions that may be the key to you conceiving, so there is no way I'm going to stop.

Ashwagandha

- Support overall endocrine system health.

Bee Pollen/Propolis

- Boosts immunity and promotes overall health.

Burdock

- Cleanses entire body.

Castor Oil

- Promotes healing and enhances circulation.

Dong Quai

- Balances hormones.

Fo-ti

- An adaptogen (works with adrenal system to balance hormones).

Ginger

- Improves overall health including that of your eggs.

Lemon Balm

- Lessens stress, depression, and anxiety which can prevent production of health eggs.

Maca

- Supports and increases egg health by protecting the body from stress damage.

Milk Thistle

- Aids liver in ridding the body of toxins which can affect egg health.

Motherwort

- Relieves those pesky symptoms of depression, anxiety, and stress.

Oat Straw/Milky Straw

- Reduces stress.

Herbs to balance progesterone levels

Proper progesterone and estrogen levels are key to conceiving. Do not continue using once pregnant.

Alfalfa

- Protects against harmful, chemically-created xenohormones.

Ashwaganda

- Support endocrine system.

Burdock

- Cleanses liver to reduce estrogen.

Eleuthero

- Necessary for proper endocrine function.

Maca

- Balances estrogen and progesterone.

- **Schisandra**

- Supports endocrine system.

Vitex

- Increases luteinizing hormone (LH) and inhibits follicle stimulating hormone (FSH) and together progesterone levels increase.

Herbs that increase sperm count and health

Guys, this section is all about you! Half the genetic makeup of your child comes from you, so make it healthy. Your health is just as important as the female's. Don't think you can get out of having to change your eating habits and supplement intake. These herbs all improve sperm quality, quantity, and motility, but they have some other functions that I think you will find beneficial.

American Ginseng

- Improves sex drive and sexual performance and treats erectile dysfunction (ED).

Ashwagandha

- Improves sex drive.

Cordyceps

- Enhance sexual function.

Edimedium

- Helps sustain an erection, increase sex drive and performance.

Fo-ti

- Treats erectile dysfunction.

Ginko

- Number one remedy for ED.

Goji Berry

- Protects sperm.

Maca

- Increases libido.

Saw Palmetto

- Improves sex drive.

Schisandra

- Reduces stress.

Tribulus

- Increases sex hormones.

Herbs that combat stress-related infertility

Stress wreaks havoc on all the body's systems, yet seems like the hardest thing to manage. Our daily lives—jobs, in-laws, our own family, finances, etc.—surround us with stress. Stress can exhaust us, and we need all our energy to have a healthy pregnancy. We need ways to replace that energy and balance our hormones so life can be enjoyed. These herbs will help. Do not continue using once pregnant.

Ashwagandha

- Re-regulates thyroid and adrenal gland function. Help endocrine system improve stress responses.

Bee Pollen/Propolis

- Helps with immunity, fertility, inflammation, and stress.

Chamomile

- Reduces stress.

Eluthero

- Strengthens immune system. Eases severe stress.

Fo-ti

- Treats stress, nervous tension, and insomnia.

Lemon Balm

- Improves stress responses and lessens depression and anxiety.

Linden

- Lowers blood pressure and reduces depression.

Maca

- Nourishing to endocrine system.

Motherwort

- Supports heart health and reduces anxiety.

Schisandra

- Supports healthy hormonal responses.

Shatavari

- Immune system and nutritive tonic.

Reishi Mushrooms

- Improves adrenal cortical function which supports the body during states of stress.

Herb to combat uterine fibroids

Uterine fibroids are considered an estrogen-dominant condition; therefore, these herbs will balance estrogen and progesterone. Uterine fibroids are also an inflammatory issue, and these herbs also act as anti-inflammatories. Do not continue using once pregnant.

Bee Propolis

- Extremely anti-inflammatory.

Black Haw

- Relaxes uterine muscles allowing for toxin removal and overall healthier uterus.

Black Cohosh

- Reduces uterine inflammation.

Blue Cohosh

- Strengthens and tones uterus.

Blue Vervain

- Supports proper uterine functions.

Castor Oil

- Helps dissolve foreign tissues like fibroids.

Cramp Bark

- Smooths uterine muscles.

Dong Quai

- Removes excess tissue growth, heals damaged tissues, limits scar tissue and adhesions.

Ginger

- Reduces inflammation.

Maca

- Supports endocrine system.

Motherwort

- Improves uterine tone.

Red Raspberry Leaf

- One of the best herbs for uterine health.

Shepherd's Purse

- Supports normal tissue growth.

Vitex

- Normalizes reproductive system.

White Peony

- Moves blood in pelvic region to lessen stagnation.

Yarrow

- Strengthens a weak uterus.

Herbs that improve overall uterine health

The muscles and lining of the uterus must be healthy to conceive, and these blood nourishing herbs can do just that.

Borage Seed Oil

- Contracts and relaxes uterine muscles.

Blue Cohosh

- Strengthens and tones uterus.

Castor Oil

- Promotes proper formation and function of uterine tissue.

Dong Quai

- Increases circulation to uterus.

Evening Primrose Oil

- Directly affects uterine cells.

Hibiscus

- Nourishes uterine lining.

Nettles

- Encourages proper tissue and blood formation.

Red Clover

- Supports proper uterine tissue development.

Red Raspberry Leaf

- Tones uterine muscles.

Did you notice a pattern in these lists? Hopefully, you noticed that many of these herbs can do double, triple, etc. duty. Herbalists can tell you which herbs will also partner well together. Some of these herbs are taken orally, and others are used as salves. There are far too many directions to list for each herb in the limited space of this book. An entire book could be dedicated to herbal remedies, and I encourage you to do research on herbs that are important to pre- and post-pregnancy health and long-term health for men, women, and children. Prescription and over-the-counter medications are not always the best answer or the first choice we should turn to. Keep this in mind – ancient civilizations have used herbs for thousands of years to treat a multitude of ailments. And none of these herbs have ever had lawsuits brought against them for causing detrimental or fatal reactions. You won't see a commercial for 1-800-BAD-HERB with a non-attorney spokesperson encouraging you to look for your portion of the compensation. Hmm¼

As I wrote this section, I realized how many natural remedies there are for my depression, anxiety, and general overall hormonal imbalances. The paragraph before this one explains how there are virtually no dangerous side effects from herbs. I could replace my prescription toxins with all-natural substances and still help my body regulate my hormones. I wouldn't have to worry about suicidal thoughts and actions, neuropsychiatric symptoms, seizure, hypertension, activation of mania or hypomania, anxiety, panic attacks, impulsivity, hostility, aggression, hyperactivity, psychosis and other neuropsychiatric reactions, and hypersensitivity reactions that are common with the two of the four medications I'm currently taking. Not to mention the lesser effects of agitation, dry mouth, insomnia, headache/migraine, nausea/vomiting, constipation, tremor, dizziness, excessive sweating, blurred vision, tachycardia, confusion, rash, hostility, cardiac arrhythmia, and auditory disturbance. So I keep asking myself why I don't wean myself off the prescriptions and try an herbal approach. After days and nights of thinking, I came up with this reason—I'm scared. I'm scared shitless. My doctors have me terrified that if I try to go off these meds, I will experience extreme symptoms of depression, anxiety, and anger that will be worse than I endured prior to starting the medication twelve years ago. I remember what I was like twelve years ago and so do my husband and daughter. They have begged me not to return to my old Jekyll and Hyde personality. I feel trapped. I chose a medical route that I don't feel I can change. But you have the ability to use a natural approach to any medical issues you may have now or in the future. If the herbal approach doesn't work to your satisfaction, you have traditional medicine to fall back on. Be brave! Don't make the same mistakes I made. Because of my choice to treat my problems with man-made solutions, I became a high risk for another pregnancy and now live with regret and fear. Live life the way nature intended—it's been around a lot longer than man.

CHAPTER THREE

COMMON STRUCTURAL AND ANATOMICAL CAUSES AND SOLUTIONS FOR INFERTILITY

There are many structural or anatomical causes for infertility in women and men. Boy, I bet men didn't realize how much of this book would apply to them. I will deal with the female concerns first.

Blocked Fallopian Tubes

One or both of the fallopian tubes can be blocked, which prevents the sperm from connecting with the egg. The blockage can be caused from hydrosalpinx—the tube fills with fluid. Tubal scarring, undetected, untreated infections (salpingitis), and past infections like Sexually Transmitted Diseases (STDs) in the tubes can also cause the blockage. And endometriosis lesions within the uterine lining are another cause. Do not assume you have blockage just because you are struggling to conceive. The only sure way to know is to have a doctor perform test called a hysterosalpingogram. Once an accurate diagnosis is made, you can make the decision of how to proceed with treatment.

If the blocked tubes are not treated, infertility is not the only concern. A fertilized egg may develop in the tube since it can't reach the uterus. This is a tubular pregnancy, and the rate of miscarriage and health risks to the mother in this situation are great. I learned this after I had surgery to cauterize my uterus. Because my uterus was now a hostile environment for a fertilized egg, the egg would grow in the fallopian tube instead. My gynecologist, whom I trusted completely, (But remember this is also the person who encouraged me to immediately look into heavy duty antipsychotics and antidepressants to cure my mood and emotional problems.) informed me that if I were to conceive after the procedure, I would have to abort the fetus. This scared the hell out of me and my husband. I don't picket or protest for prolife or prochoice, but there was no way I would abort a fetus. Needless to say, my husband and I never have unprotected sex. Even though the chances of pregnancy are slim, I don't ever want to be in that position.

Here are some natural therapies to combat fallopian tube health. Of course, using the herbs mentioned in the last chapter will benefit you, but these therapies are specific for fallopian tube abnormalities. You should consult and work directly with an herbalist or all-natural medical practitioner to help administer these treatments. **All of these treatments are meant to be used prior to conception**.

The first treatment is a fertility cleansing. This cleansing will give your body a clean slate on which other herbs and treatment will benefit from. This cleansing is not just aimed at the reproductive system. The liver is also important to cleanse due to its ability to balance hormones and remove toxins from the body. This cleanse will also improve circulation to the reproductive system. This circulation will help remove stagnant blood which creates an unhealthy environment for an embryo. Because this cleanse is done prior to pregnancy, anyone can benefit from it. This cleanse should be done about one month prior to trying to conceive because the herbs used are not recommended for use once pregnant. Even if your fallopian tubes are healthy, a cleanse will create the healthiest, safest environment for a growing fetus.

A fertility cleanse does more for the reproductive system than a whole body cleanse. This is because a fertility cleanse works with the menstrual cycle. This type of cleanse uses whole herbs, while other cleanses use teas, powders, drinks, etc. A fertility cleanse uses less astringent herbs. Some of the herbs that are used are burdock, milk thistle seed, dandelion root, yellow dock root (stimulates bile production), licorice root, ginger root, goldenseal root (anti-inflammatory used to prevent scar tissue and adhesion formation), damiana leaf (increases circulation to reproductive system), dong quai, peony root, and raspberry leaf. Some women "feel" the cleanse working, while others wonder if it is working. It is working whether you fell different or not. Your body's reaction has to do with your previous diet and exposure to environmental toxins. Since this cleanse cannot hurt you, give it a try!

Another method to consider is systematic enzyme therapy. This method specifically targets excess tissue, especially scar tissue. It also cleanses the blood (fresh oxygenated, free-flowing blood promotes egg health), reduces inflammation, eases minor pain, and improves circulation to the reproductive system. This therapy's ability to combat excess tissue is vital. Excess tissue is a common reason for poor fallopian health. Systematic enzymes also regulate the immune system and possibly prevent recurrent miscarriages.

A third therapy is abdominal or fertility massages. These increase circulation and break up adhesions. These massages should be performed by massage therapists who specialize in fertility massage. The most common benefits from this type of therapy are: unblocking fallopian tubes, breaking up scar tissue, increasing circulation, reducing inflammation, and loosening tight or twisted tissues.

Castor oil therapy is done externally with the use of packs placed on the abdominal region. As the body absorbs the oil, circulation to the reproductive system increases and the lymphatic system begins removing waste like old diseased cells and tissues.

The fifth and final therapy is herbal. An herbal treatment does four key things: reduces inflammation, promotes healthy circulation, reduces infection, and supports hormonal balance. The following herbs are used in alone and in combination for this treatment; therefore, consulting an herbalist is important in order to achieve optimal results: goldenseal, ginger root, dong quai, hawthorn (reduces abdominal congestion), peony root, wild yam, and uva ursi (reduces congestion and fluid retention).

Hydrosalpinx

This is commonly caused by untreated STDs, especially gonorrhea and chlamydia, IUDs, endometriosis, and abdominal surgery. The damage causes the end of the fallopian tube to close and fluid to collect. This fluid is toxic and can flush the embryo out of the uterus. The same therapies are used to treat his problem as the ones used to treat blocked fallopian tubes.

Ovarian Cysts

I know from experience that ovarian cysts are painful. I was taken to the emergency room in college because I thought the intense pain in my abdomen and lower back was caused by my appendix. This pain was so bad that it hurt to go to the bathroom, walk, and even sit down. After much time and some uncomfortable prodding and probing, the doctor informed me I had ovarian cysts and to follow up with my gynecologist. Well, you'll never guess what his solution was—birth control pills. He didn't even examine me. He just walked in the room, shook my hand, and handed me a one-month supply of the pill. Just another example of a medical professional turning to medication first as a solution to a common problem. Being sexually active and definitely not ready to be a parent, I jumped on the chance to start the pill. After less than a month, I had to take myself off the pill. I was suicidal; I would actually contemplate going full speed into telephone poles, concrete embankments, and bridge supports. Thankfully, I read the side effects of the pill and realized what was causing my daredevil driving. I experience painful cysts on rare occasions, but when I do, I bear with the pain and give a nod of gratitude for my wonderful life. The morning after writing this paragraph I woke up to painful cysts. Talk about power of suggestion.

Ovarian cysts are usually benign and painless, but they can cause fertility problems. A dermoid cyst can become inflamed and cause ovarian torsion (twisting). An endometrioid cyst is caused by a common fertility problem—endometriosis. Polycystic ovary syndrome (PCOS) also causes infertility. There are other varieties of ovarian cysts, but all can be treated with natural therapies.

The first step is to reduce estrogen by avoiding exposure to xenoestrogens. To successfully do this, you need to stop eating all soy products, eat only organic meats and dairy products, and stop drinking water that has been bottled in plastic. You should also avoid mineral oil and parabens in skin care products and use only all-natural detergents. It's amazing to me how many toxins are absorbed into the body through the skin.

The second step is to increase progesterone and balance hormones. Excess estrogen creates a deficiency in progesterone. A balance between the two is necessary for conception. The common treatment is to use progesterone cream under the guidance of an herbalist or medical professional. The following herbs are used to balance hormones: maca root, black cohosh root, dong quai, milk thistle seed, tribulus, vitex, wild yam root, and yarrow.

The third step is to dissolve and reduce the cysts. The ways to do this are systematic enzyme therapy and castor oil packs. Sound familiar?

Fibroid Tumors

These are some doozies. They can be benign and non-problematic or they can cause infertility and recurrent miscarriages. Common factors that cause fibroid tumors are expended periods of excess estrogen in the body, exposure to xenoestrogens (eat organic foods, avoid exposure to pesticides, herbicides, synthetic fertilizers and plastics, use organic body care and makeup products, do not ingest preservatives and dyes, use low VOC [volatile organic compound] paints, use recycled unbleached paper products and non-chlorinated laundry bleach), poor metabolism, hypertension, complications from IUDs perineal talc use, cycles without ovulation, and PCOS. The "traditional" method of dealing with these tumors if they are causing fertility issues is surgical procedures. This is not the only course of action.

First perform a cleanse like the one used to combat blocked fallopian tubes. Eat more dark leafy green, broccoli, swiss chard, quinoa, chia seeds, beans, and ground flaxseed.

Step two is to increase circulation with herbs. Pau d'arco (an antibacterial), goldenseal root, dandelion root and leaf, ginger root, black cohosh root, red raspberry leaf, dong quia, and maitake mushrooms (enhances immune system) are all suggested herbs. Fertility massage and castor oil packs will also increase circulation.

A third consideration is systematic enzyme therapy. I feel like I've written that before.

Autoimmune Diseases that Can Affect Fertility

Dr. Norbert Gleicher defines autoimmune disease as, "a varied group of over 80 serious, chronic illnesses that affect almost every human organ system." When the body's autoimmune system is malfunctioning, the body can begin fighting itself and affect connective tissues that bind various tissues and organs. The endocrine system, essential for proper reproductive health, is an area that will be under attack. These conditions may be genetic, hormonal, or environmental.

The following diseases affect the nervous system: multiple sclerosis, myasthenia gravis, autoimmune neuropathies, Guillain-Barre, and autoimmune uveitis.

The following autoimmune diseases affect the endocrine glands: type 1/immune mediated diabetes mellitus, grave's disease, hashimoto's thyroiditis, autoimmune oophoritis/orchitis, autoimmune adrenal diseases.

The following are autoimmune diseases that affect the blood vessels: anti-phospholipid antibody syndrome, temporal arteritis, vasculitides, Wegener's granulumatosis, and Behcet's disease.

Of course there are many other forms of autoimmune diseases. I am concentrating on the ones which affect fertility the most. Dr. Weil from Weil Health Centers recommends combating all autoimmune diseases with these dietary changes:

Reduce protein intake to ten percent of total calories; replace animal protein as much as possible with plant protein. Eliminate milk and milk products (substitute other calcium sources). Eat ore fruits and vegetables (make sure they are all organically grown). Eliminate polyunsaturated vegetable oils, margarine, vegetable shortening, all partially hydrogenated oils, and all foods (such as deep-fried foods) that might contain trans-fatty acids. Use extra-virgin olive oil as your main fat. Increase your intake of omega-3 fatty acids. Eat plenty of foods high in potassium, such as oranges, tomatoes, apricots and their juices, bananas, and broccoli. Ginger and turmeric are herbs that can be taken to reduce flare-ups and inflammation.

Each disease is defined in this book's Glossary of Terms, so here I will discuss how it affects fertility and what natural ways are used to treat it. Unfortunately, some of these diseases are seriously complicated and have not been successfully treated by natural means.

The nervous system is in control of all the body's functions and systems. The central nervous system send signals to all parts of the body, and if those signals are interfered with or don't reach their intended target, the entire body can be affected.

There is no scientific proof that multiple sclerosis (MS) impairs fertility. Some women have feared that getting pregnant could worsen their MS symptoms, but many women over the years have experienced reduced MS relapses. Pregnancy increases the number of circulating proteins that act as natural immunosuppressants. Pregnancy also increases natural corticosteroid levels which can lessen the symptoms of multiple sclerosis.

Myasthenia gravis causes weakening in muscles, but it does not affect fertility. Some women do not experience any changes in their symptoms during pregnancy, while others experienced a worsening of symptoms. There is no medical rhyme or reason for these drastic differences in experiences. Remember doctors "practice" medicine; they haven't perfected anything. Myasthenia gravis does not impair the growth and development of the fetus, thus there are no higher risks of birth defects. Good news!

Autoimmune neuropathies can affect the communication of the central nervous system and the reproductive system. When this occurs, movement of certain muscles in that area are affected. Some rare but serious affects are muscle wasting, paralysis, and/ or organ or gland dysfunction. The body may be unable to digest food easily, maintain safe levels of blood pressure, sweat normally, and/or experience normal sexual function. Acupuncture is the most common drug-free treatment for neuropathies.

Guillain-Barre causes weakness or paralysis and extreme fatigue; therefore, a substantial recovery period (at least twelve months) should pass before considering pregnancy. Treating the symptoms as early as possible will reduce long-term effects. Medical treatments can be one of these two – a plasma exchange or immunoglobulin therapy. Thankfully, Ashwagandha is an herb that is effective in reducing the paralysis symptoms of Guillain-Barre syndrome. Bala or country mallow aids in healing all the symptoms of the disease, especially paralysis, and it strengthens limbs and improves the circulatory system. Ginger can ease the symptoms by providing essential nutrients to the body. Nux vomica or kuchla has proven effective in treating the paralysis associated with Guillain-Barre syndrome. And tribulus eases the symptoms. After excessive research, I was unable to find proof that Guillain-Barre syndrome causes fertility problems. Yea!

Autoimmune uveitis is an inflammatory disease that affects the eye. Since this does not affect pregnancy or fertility, I will move on.

The endocrine system is essential for hormonal health, especially sexual function and reproduction. And one autoimmune disease affected by this system is type 1 diabetes. Women and men can experience sexual dysfunction from diabetes. Women sexual problems include reduced sensation is genitals, dryness, difficulty/inability to orgasm, pain during sex, and decreased libido. Women can experience problems with their menstrual cycle. Such as oligomenorrhea (very light or infrequent periods) and secondary amenorrhea (absence of periods). Amenorrhea can be naturally treated with saffron and milk (not cow's milk), soaked chickpeas mixed with jiggery, eating spinach, parsley, and flaxseed, increase your zinc intake through the foods you eat, and tomato juice mixed with fennel and cinnamon. Diabetes in any form should be monitored under the supervision of a health care professional. None of the sexually related effects of type 1 diabetes causes infertility. If you follow the directions of your doctor, you can have a successful conception and pregnancy.

Men's sexual dysfunctions include erectile dysfunction and ejaculation that sends the sperm to the man's bladder instead of into the female reproductive system. Two important lifestyle changes to make with type 1 diabetes are proper diet and daily exercise. Specifically, the man's diet should regulate his carbohydrate intake. This sexual dysfunctions are not debilitating for fertility; therefore, treating the symptoms and maintaining a healthy diet and exercise regimen will result in the ability to fertilize your partner's egg.

Grave's disease in women necessitates the need for a serious discussion and then decision when considering pregnancy. The fetus will be at risk, but there are no means in which to monitor the effects. Make sure the symptoms are under control before getting pregnant or taking the steps to become pregnant. But even this does not guarantee a healthy fetus. Grave's disease affects the thyroid and can cause hyperthyroidism and hypothyroidism in the fetus. Thankfully, there are natural ways to try and control the symptoms like flaxseed oil, broccoli, bugleweed, radishes, and kelp. This serious condition does require the help and guidance of medical professionals.

Hashimoto's thyroiditis affects the thyroid function. Five of the most natural ways to combat the symptoms of this thyroid problem are pranaya, walnuts, kelp, coconut oil, and fish oil. Pranaya is actually a yogic breathing exercise. You sit cross-legged on the floor, a cushion, or mat, and placed your hands on your knees with your palms facing upward. You will breathe in fully through your nose while inflating the abdomen. Then exhale through your nose while contracting the stomach muscles and trying to press them toward your spine. Doing this for fifteen minutes a day will help remove toxins from your body, relieve tension and stress, and teach you deep breathing that will be helpful during labor and delivery.

Oophotitis/orchitis is an inflammation of the ovaries. It can be seen in conjunction with salpingitis which is an inflammation of the fallopian tubes. Both of these conditions can cause fertility issues in women. In the case of oophotitis, the ovaries may become damaged and result in the inability to produce an egg or a health egg. Oophotitis is commonly treated with antibiotics, and when it has gone untreated or misdiagnosed more drastic medical procedures like a hysterectomy are performed. Much less invasive treatments include massage and chiropractic. Black berry or jambul, drumstick flowers, amla, dates, and cottage cheese are natural foods and herbs to promote ovarian health. But I would recommend seeking medical advise when treating oophotitis since leaving it untreated may require a hysterectomy.

Common symptoms of adrenal diseases include but are not limited to weakness, fatigue, anorexia, nausea, vomiting, constipation, diarrhea, abdominal pain, salt cravings, and postural dizziness. When trying to conceive, your body should not be experiencing any of these symptoms; therefore, you must address and treat these symptoms as soon as possible. Your adrenal gland regulates blood pressure, energy levels, immune function, and all processes that handle stress. We know that stress is one of the biggest culprits of infertility, so adrenal gland health is of utmost importance. Here are some natural ways to combat the symptoms of adrenal diseases: almonds, figs, bananas, citrus fruit, green tea, and beet juice. Herbs like scutellaria lateriflora, rhodiola rosea, Ashwagandha, Siberian ginseng, changxan, licorice, and cordycep will all help improve adrenal health.

Blood vessel disorders can affect fertility because proper blood flow to all systems and organs in the body is essential for optimal health. I know you've read repeatedly in this book about blood flow and its importance. You understand why it's important, and I know you will take the necessary steps to combat the symptoms and diseases of improper blood flow. So without further ado...

Anti-phospholipid antibody syndrome causes the body to destroy normal proteins in the blood. This can cause blood clots, miscarriage, and stillbirth. Major organs can also be affects like the kidney, heart, and lungs. There is no cure for this disease. But there ways to reduce your risks of blood clots. Natural ways to prevent blood clots from forming are to keep moving, drink lots of water, avoid birth control pills and hormone replacement therapy (HRT), and get regular heart checkups. Once blood clots have formed, here are some natural ways to treat them: drink lots of water, hot and cold compresses alternately applied to the site of the blood clot, get plenty of Vitamin C, Vitamin E, and omega-3 fatty acids. Ingesting fibrin-rich foods and herbs on a daily basis like onions, garlic, turmeric, ginger, bilberry, gingko, and cayenne. You also need foods rich in folate. Folate can be found in bread, beans, asparagus, Brussels sprouts, whole meal cereals, broccoli, spinach, and cloves. Walking and yoga are perfect activities to treat blood clots.

Temporal arteritis is a serious condition when the blood vessels that supply blood to the head are inflamed, swollen, and/or tender. Treatment most begin immediately after being diagnosed, so natural, home treatments are not recommended. Medline Plus states that if you experience any of these symptoms, seek treatment immediately:

throbbing headache on one side of the head or the back of the head, tenderness when touching the scalp, excessive sweating, fever, general ill feeling, jaw pain that comes and goes or occurs when chewing, loss of appetite, muscle aches, pain and stiffness in the neck, upper arms, shoulder, and hips, weakness, excessive tiredness, blurred vision, double vision, or reduce vision in one or both eyes. You may also experience bleeding gums, face pain, hearing loss, and joint stiffness.

Holy crap! I used to experience some of those symptoms after a night of hard drinking. But stupidity aside, that's a lot of things that a person can feel that may or may not have anything to do blood flow. How's a person to know? The more aware you are of your body and the healthier you are, the easier it will be for you to notice changes that are serious enough to address with a doctor.

Vasculitides or vasculitis causes a change in the walls of the blood vessels. These changes can be a thickening, weakening, narrowing, and scarring. This is a very rare condition but is treatable by controlling inflammation. Mayo Clinic lists the following as common signs and symptoms: fever, headache, fatigue, weight loss, general aches and pains, night sweats, rashes, nerve problems like numbness or weakness, and/or the loss of a pulse in a limb. Complications can include organ damage, blood clots and aneurysms, vision loss or blindness, and infections like pneumonia and blood infections. A traditional doctor will begin a regimen of prescription drugs. There are natural ways to keep your blood vessels healthy from the start and they are regular exercise, healthy diet that includes cayenne pepper, ginger root, garlic, Gingko Biloba Goji berries, watermelon, and dark chocolate. Take hot showers, get massages, quit smoking, wear comfortable shoes, find an acupuncturist, and meditate.

Another blood vessel condition is Wegener's granulumatosis. This condition inflames the blood vessels and restricts blood flow to vital areas of the body like kidneys, lungs, skin, eyes, ears, spinal cord, heart and upper respiratory tract. Traditional medicine will prescribe medications that may lower your body's ability to fight infections. In fact, one type of drug used for treatment is from the immune suppressant branch of medicines. When thinking about treating inflammatory conditions consider using arnica, white willow bark, boswellia, devil's claw, turmeric, bromelain, ginger, burdock, flax, nettles, licorice.

The final autoimmune disease I will cover is Behcet's disease. This disease inflames the blood vessels throughout the body. Signs of the disease are mouth sores, eye inflammation, skin rashes and lesions, as well as genital sores. There is no cure for Behcet's disease, but doctors can treat it with things such a skin creams, gels, or ointments, mouth rinses, and eyedrops. The following foods can help combat inflammation throughout the body: olive oil, garlic, turmeric, ginger, salmon, cherries, sweet potatoes, spinach, walnuts, and blueberries.

Uterine Abnormalities

Some women are born with abnormalities of the uterus. These can be a double uterus, a uterus where only one side has fully developed, and uterine septum (a tissue "wall" dividing the uterus). These do not automatically result in infertility, so don't panic.

Unfortunately, I was unable to find natural ways to combat the complications these abnormalities cause. In these cases, consult your doctor or midwife.

Causes of male infertility

Sexually Transmitted Diseases

A huge cause of infertility is past sexually transmitted diseases. Back when sex education could be taught in schools, I knew a middle school principal who decided to take a drastic approach to teach the eighth grade boys and girls about STDs. First, he didn't separate the boys and the girls. His philosophy was they contract it together, they should learn about it together. Next, thanks to a friend in the medical field, he showed actual, up-close photos of male and female infections. I'm not sure how effective this approach was since a follow-up study was never done. (Why do I get the impression the first time those kids had sex, they had those graphic images in their heads?) But give some serious thought about the moments of sexual gratification during unprotected sex versus painful and damaging STDs that can haunt you for a lifetime.

Lifestyle Factors

The following factors temporarily affect the sperm quality and motility. All of these factors are combatable if you are truly willing to impregnate your partner.

- Testicular overheating

- Substance Abuse

- Smoking

- Obesity

- Bicycling

- Emotional Stress

Environmental Factors

Intense exposure to certain chemicals, toxins, or heavy metals can cause fertility problems. But this exposure needs to be chronic and long-term in order to create irreversible damage.

Medical Conditions

The following are medical reasons for infertility and natural ways to combat them:

- Severe injury to genital area – For men aged thirty-five and younger, herbal therapies have been found to help restore the penis to pre-injury health. Here are the suggested herbs: alisma plantago (accelerates healing), astragalus membranaceus (stimulates immune system to speed recovery), cistanche (improves blood circulation to reproductive system), curculigo (enhances penile erection and increases sperm count), eurycoma longifolia (produces more testosterone), maca, morinda (energizes sexual organs), panax ginseng (improves sexual nervous system), rhodiola (restores malfunctioning biological systems), sarsaparilla Jamaican (increases testosterone), schisandra, and tribulus.

- Diabetes – can cause retrograde ejaculation (semen backs up into bladder) which prevents the sperm from reaching the female reproductive organs. Diabetes in men can cause DNA damage which will be transferred to the egg and may cause fetal deformities. Herbs to combat high glucose levels are: Ashwagandha, cinnamon, and burdock.

- HIV – Because of the severity of HIV and the possibility of transmitting the disease to your partner and unborn child, this issue should be handled by a medical professional.

- Thyroid disease – Your diet should include raw cranberries, whole fat yogurt, raw dairy products, navy beans, strawberries, potatoes with the skin, and Himalayan crystal salt. Ashwagandha and rhodiola are two herbs that support a healthy endocrine system.

- Cushing syndrome – This is an endocrine disorder that produces too much cortisol causing men to have a decline in sperm production. Ginseng is the most common herb used to treat Cushing syndrome symptoms.

- Heart attack – Sperm production can be impaired after a heart attack. Consider using ginseng to boost production.

- Liver and/or kidney failure – The problem and suggested remedy for liver and kidney failure matches that of a heart attack.

- Chronic anemia – Should be treated like a heart attack or liver or kidney failure.

- Infections in the urinary tract and/or genitals – After an infection, there is potential for scar tissue. Using a castor oil pack can reduce tissue inflammation and growth.

- Cancer and any of its treatments – Chemotherapy and radiation can severely impair sperm production. Try ginseng to combat this condition.

All afore mentioned conditions will affect sperm quality, quantity, and motility. Without the male part of the equation there is no chance for a baby. Even if a man is not considering parenthood in the near future, he can still benefit from this information. Young people often think they are invincible and don't realize the long-term effects their actions in their teens and twenties can have. Don't hesitate – educate. To correct sperm count, swimming ability, and overall quality, please see the list of herbs that can aid in these improvements. Think of it this way, if you have a high-performance vehicle, you're not going to take risks with it. You'll use only high-quality oil that is engineered for cars of that caliber. No low- or mid-grade fuel that could clog up the engine with impurities. You don't park it near other cars in a parking lot; you usually take up three spaces by parking on an odd angle so no one can damage the body. If you take this much care and concern with a vehicle, shouldn't you treat your sperm with as much if not more. Think about it, your sperm is your way of giving life to someone who can carry on your legacy. But more importantly, your sperm will help create one of the most miraculous events in your life.

Structural Abnormalities

Hypospadias is a birth defect that causes the urinary opening to be on the underside of the penis. Cryptorchidism is a condition in which a testicle does not descend from the abdomen into the scrotum. And blockage in the tubes that transport the sperm is another abnormality that can affect fertility. All three conditions impair sperm production and transportation but does not mean pregnancy is out of the question. Using the herbs listed to increase sperm production and health should be your first course of action. These herbs are: ginseng and tribulus.

CHAPTER FOUR

ACUPUNCTURE

Many reputable western medical specialists are recognizing the benefits some patients experience with acupuncture. Some highly respected clinics through the United States are incorporating acupuncture with traditional medicine. My husband and I had to unfortunately pay a visit to the best neurological surgical center in Chicago, Illinois. I was shocked to find an acupuncturist's office directly across the hall from the surgeon's consultation waiting room. I realized then the profound impact ancient practices can have in modern times. Acupuncture is an ancient form of treatment for the body's ailments that has been used for over 5000 years. It involves in insertion of sterilized needles into specific points on the body. The needles are rarely felt as they are inserted because they are barely thicker than a human hair. The needles are inserted in the body's channels or meridians (which form a grid pattern on the body from head to toe) which help regulate various body functions. The Ancient Chinese believed that the body contains two opposing and inseparable forces: yin and yang. Yin represents the cold, slow, or passive principle. The yang represents the hot, excited, or active principle. These two principles must be in alignment for Qi to flow properly. According to James Dillard MD, the points the needles enter are considered "'energy points' believed to regulate spiritual, mental, emotional, and physical balance." Acupuncture stimulates your body's Qi or life energy that needs to freely flow through your body at all times. And your Qi needs to be calm, balanced throughout the body, and fully restored (in other words-reduce stress) in order to accept the creation of life. In the nineteenth century, a common procedure to treat disease was bloodletting. Physicians of the time believed that illness was present in the blood, so removing the infected blood would essentially heal the patient. This practice worked on rare occasions but was eventually banned. In today's medical world, some diseases require blood transfusions and dialysis to cleanse the blood, but bloodletting is no longer used. The fact that acupuncture started before bloodletting and continues today, just amazes me.

If you can't quite wrap your head around the idea of QI, then maybe this will help—acupuncture also stimulates the brain to produce endorphins which regulate the menstrual cycle. The brain will work with the hypothalamus and pituitary glands and the ovaries to impact egg production and a healthy ovulation. The needles also promote blood flow which is vital for proper organ function. Acupuncture during pregnancy should only be done under the care of an acupuncturist trained in this area. Some places the needles are inserted should be avoided once pregnant. Insertion pf the needles in certain places could stimulate labor and cause premature labor. Make sure you double and triple check the ability of your acupuncturist to work with you once pregnant. Mayo Clinic recommends you look to people you trust for recommendations of practitioners. Check that the practitioner has finished all training and earned all certifications. Lastly, interview the practitioner. Get all your questions and concerns answered to your satisfaction. No question is too little or silly. This is your health and the health of your potential unborn child. You must literally trust this person with your life.

During your first visit to an acupuncturist, they will examine the following: any areas where you are experiencing pain, the shape, coating, and color of your tongue, the color of your face, and the strength, rhythm, and quality of the pulse in your wrist. Once the insertion of the needles begins, you may question where the needles are being placed in relation to the area you have requested be treated. Acupuncture points are located all over the body, and can affect areas not even close to where the needles are being inserted. The human body is amazing. Did you know that certain points on you r feet can cause you to lose consciousness? Some people experience a mild aching sensation when the needle reaches the correct depth. Then the practitioner may move the needles in a twisting manner or apply heat or mild electrical pulses to the needles. The needles will remain inserted for about ten to twenty minutes, and you will not experience pain when the needles are removed. During the treatment session, some practitioners will talk to you about ways to heal yourself through diet and exercise. And they may also encourage a different model for thinking about your health.

In the case of fertility, acupuncture can help regulate under- (hypothyroidism) and over-active (hyperthyroidism) thyroid issues that may be causing problems. It can treat disorders caused by spasms in the fallopian tubes. It can also treat elevated follicle stimulation hormone (FSH), recurrent miscarriage, unexplained (idiopathic) infertility, luteal phase defect, hyperprolactinemia (not caused by prolactinoma), and polycystic ovarian syndrome with annovulatory cycles. Men with sperm-DNA-fragmentation will also benefit from acupuncture. Sperm health will significantly improve and sperm count and motility might also improve. Acupuncture is also used as a natural painkiller for menstrual cramps and labor pain. The body's neuroendocrine system will be activated to release hormones that stimulate the ovaries, the adrenal glands, and other reproductive organs and systems. Acupuncture also reduces the stress caused by infertility. And reducing stress is key for a healthy life.

Acupuncture cannot help all areas of fertility concern. But if it is coupled with herbal treatments, the two can combat several issues. Together they can improve ovarian and follicle function and increase blood flow to the endometrium. Unfortunately, acupuncture cannot treat tubal adhesions which can occur from pelvic inflammatory disease (PID) or endometriosis. It also cannot treat blocked fallopian tubes. But look back in the herbal section of this book to find several herbs that can help reduce adhesions and promote the body's natural defenses against adhesions forming. Men can also benefit from acupuncture to help their fertility issues. Acupuncture can be used in conjunction with other fertility treatments. You may have a higher success rate if using more than one treatment to combat your issues.

Just like with herbal treatments, acupuncture should begin well before the woman becomes pregnant. Acupuncture is not a one-time-fix-all approach. Instead it is an on-going procedure that over time will help in areas of fertility. There is no magic cure for the problems women and men go through when trying to conceive. Remember you cannot be considered infertile until one year of actively trying to conceive has passed. Nature can't be rushed.

Someone needs to tell the farmers who are adding hormones to our foods to rush nature's growth cycle that Mother Nature has a plan and don't mess with it! Advances in science can be lifesaving and healing, but our bodies aren't meant to ingest absorb foreign substances. Carefully consider natural versus medical treatments. I feel like I've said that before.

Make sure you do research into acupuncturists in your area and make sure the one you choose specializes in fertility acupuncture. The wonderful thing about trying acupuncture is that you are not doing any damage to your body. There are virtually no risks to the patient and no long-term side effects. However, it is important to note that acupuncture does not work for everyone. It continues to amaze me that all things natural have no detrimental effects on our bodies, yet every time we turn around, we hear about another drug recall. Just listen to an advertisement for drugs and all the side effects. Look at the lengthy one to two page list of warnings in a magazine ad for medication. Why don't more people opt for natural treatments? Myself included.

CHAPTER FIVE

CHIROPRACTIC TREATMENTS

Your spine connects your brain to the rest of your body. Encased in your spine are all the nerves needed for healthy organ and other bodily functions. Chiropractors work to ensure the spine is properly aligned so there is no spinal nerve stress. Just like any other part of our body, stress is detrimental to our overall health. Stress on the nerves in our spine can cause a multitude of problems with other parts of our body. Other joints like hips and knees will hurt, and we believe the problem lies in those joints when it may actually be a result of a nerve in the spinal column. The American Pregnancy Association describes chiropractic treatments as the ability to enhance the function of the "Master Control System of the body, the nervous system."

The American Pregnancy Association suggests that when choosing a chiropractor to work with, look for the following designations:

DACC – Diplomate with International Chiropractic Pediatric Association (ICPA) reflecting highest level of advanced training

CACCP – Certified with the ICPA reflecting advanced training

Member of ICPA – reflecting special interest

Webster Certified – trained to specifically work with breech positions

Chiropractic treatment can begin before pregnancy, continue throughout the pregnancy if the chiropractor has one or more of the above designations, and can be continued post-pregnancy.

The central nervous system is in charge of the entire body and all its functions, including reproduction. Chiropractors specialize in the health of the nervous system and are able to understand how a misaligned spine can affect reproduction. Jessica Shelley provides this explanation of the chiropractic adjustment's specific effect on reproduction:

> Spinal movement contributes to the proper flow of cerebrospinal fluid (CSF). Restrictions of spinal movement alter the flow of CSF and may impact the hypothalamus and/or the pituitary gland. These glands are responsible for reproducing hormones such as follicle-stimulating hormone

and lutenizing hormone which are vital to reproductive function.

She also stated that vertebral misalignments or subluxations can affect other glands and organs that are important to proper reproductive functions. Chiropractic can help normalize the menstrual cycle by stimulating ovulation. Misalignments cause interference between the peripheral nervous system and the central nervous system. This improper nerve flow can result in the egg being unable to reach its destination for fertilization.

If your spine is properly aligned, your central nervous system will operate correctly, and your overall health and mental well-being will be positively impacted. Mental health is an important aspect of conceiving which is so often overlooked. Your goal is to eventually provide your unborn child with a safe, healthy environment in which to grow. Well, that health and safety begins before conception by treating anxiety and stress in our daily lives and associated with infertility. Stress prevents the nervous system from functioning to its full potential. Chiropractic can even promote the body's communication on a cellular level; the nervous and endocrine systems working with the reproductive system. The three systems must work in harmony, and stress interferes with that harmony. Keeping these three systems working properly should be a concern during our pre-pregnancy stage and throughout our lives.

If we can learn to handle stress better, imagine how much happier our lives would be, how much better our relationships would be, and how much more peaceful the world in general would be.

CHAPTER SIX

PREGNANCY AFTER 40

Women in their early forties are still capable of conceiving naturally. We all have our own reasons why we wait to get pregnant, and no one, especially a busy-body mother, should judge us. Stand strong in the face of pressure, Ladies. If you're not dating, people find it acceptable to ask why you don't have a man in your life. Answer—none of your business. If you are married are secure in a long-term relationship, you will be hounded about when you're going to get pregnant. "Oh, a baby would complete you." "You don't know what you're missing." "Your life isn't complete until you've felt that baby grow and kick inside you." Do you feel like kicking another part of that person's anatomy? I don't know when it became acceptable in our society to enquire freely about people's personal business. My response in these types of situations is to smile, nod, and move far, far away from that person. You'll have to find your own method of quieting people. But please remember how these questions made you feel and never do the same to some other poor woman.

Even though you still have a twenty percent chance of natural conception in your early forties, there are still some risks and things you need to understand. First, you are still producing eggs, but their quality is not what it used to be. Don't worry, they're not past their expiration date, they might just need a boost. Reread the herb lists. There are plenty of herbs that promote healthier eggs.

Secondly, there is also a chance that the eggs you now produce may contain chromosomal abnormalities. According to the CVS Pharmacy website, women who conceive in their early twenties have a 1 in 500 chance of abnormalities and a 1 in 1500 chance of conceiving a child with Down 's syndrome. Women in their late twenties have a 1 in 385 chance for abnormalities and 1 in 1100 chance for Down's. Throughout the thirties, a woman has a 1 in 178 chance of a chromosomal abnormality and a 1 in 350 chance of Down's. After forty, the chances increases to 1 in 63 for abnormalities and 1 in 25 for a child with Down syndrome. (I found other statistics with different ratios. I decided to give you one set and allow you to determine if you wanted to search for other statistics.) I felt it was important to mention this serious concern and the statistics to better explain it. Does this mean you don't try after forty? No. You just need to be aware of your risks, be positive you and your partner are willing to take the risks, and that you both are ready to love and treasure a child who may have birth defects. Here's a positive statistic, after 45 you have a one in two chance of having twins!

I know several women who conceived in their forties. All the children were healthy, but their obstetrician told them they had to have all the tests and procedures like amniocentesis and repeated ultrasounds. They all followed their doctors' orders. Here is my school of thought, and please take this with a grain of salt because it is just an opinion. What if a test comes back positive for chromosomal abnormalities? Are you willing to abort the fetus? What about the chances of a false positive? What about the immense stress you are going to put on yourself and your baby by worrying about the test and its results? When these tests were offered to me, I declined all of them, including the ultrasounds. I think I am the only woman who has been pregnant since the 1990s who didn't have at least one ultrasound during her pregnancy. I actually chose my obstetrician because she didn't recommend ultrasounds. My philosophy was, if the baby is born with birth defects, I will love that baby with my whole heart regardless, and I refused to put the extra stress on myself and the baby. This is just something to chew on.

Women in their forties will need to be under the care of a medical professional, obstetrician, or midwife. Because there are so many possible complications, you will need more frequent checkups. Your doctor or midwife will be as concerned about your health as they are about the health of the fetus. An unhealthy mother or one who is stressed and anxious does not provide the healthiest of conditions for the growing and developing fetus. Yes, your chances for a problematic pregnancy are twice as high as that of a woman in her twenties or early thirties. Yes, you may experience a more difficult delivery than a younger woman. But if the desire to become pregnant is more important to you and your partner than these risks, you should not hesitate to try to conceive. Many things in life come with risks that we weigh, think long and hard about, and decide to go ahead and do. As long as you're not heading into pregnancy uninformed and on a whim, this is probably the best risk you could ever take.

Just as younger women do, you should begin to immediately adjust your lifestyle, exercise routine, and diet. You will want to be in the best physical condition possible. Make sure all existing conditions are stable. These include but are not limited to high blood pressure, diabetes, thyroid disease, and obesity. Begin taking folic acid to help prevent neural tube defects, especially spina bifida. As mentioned earlier in the book, folic acid can also prevent congenital heart defects, cleft lip, limb defects, and urinary tract anomalies. Folic acid can be found in many foods

After Thoughts

I learned an incredible amount of information on health that can apply to a person looking to improve fertility or one just looking to improve overall health and wellness. However, I am not a health care specialist or professional or an herbalist or natural practitioner, nor do I play one on TV. I am not an expert in this field, so if you have concerns or questions after reading anything in this book, seek a professional. I cannot stress that enough! Yes, I did research and tried to use the most up-to-date information and reliable sources, but this does not ensure 100% accuracy or answers to your specific problems. My hope is that this book will inspire you to improve your lifestyle and diet now so you, your partner, and children will live happily and healthily ever after!

This is not my first go organic, be healthier rodeo. I have been part of other detoxification books, organic blogs, etc. My neighbor and best friend has gone completely organic with her family. She is constantly telling me how easy it is to make the changes, especially since I do all the grocery shopping and cooking. Even though this book focuses on fertility, and I am beyond needing help in that area, the research for this book reminded me of how important healthy eating and exercise is throughout our entire lives. After a project like this, I will get on my soapbox and rant to my husband and daughter about our poor eating habits, the extra weight we all carry, and our general lack of energy. They nod their heads, listen half-heartedly, and roll their eyes when I turn my back. I run out to the library and check out every whole food, raw food, and farm to table recipe book available. Shoot, I've even requested books from libraries fifty miles away! Then I go to the all-organic grocery store and spend twice as much on a week's worth of groceries. I'm all geared up. I clean all processed food out of the fridge and pantry. I silently curse my dietary weaknesses and vow to really change this time. Usually within a week, I find a reason to go back to old ways. I blame it on the cost of organic foods. I say I'm too busy to cook healthy every night, and pizza is just easier and faster. I had a craving. I've eaten these chemically altered foods my entire adult life and so far I have no negative effects. As you can tell, I can make lots of excuses and not many commitments.

There there's the whole exercise idea. I'm better in this area, but not by much. I'll join a gym and stick with it for about a month. Once I even kept my gym regimen up for three months! But then work got busy. I tried bicycling and loved it. Unfortunately, I live in a part of the country where the bike riding season lasts for four months at most. And after spending each ride in the beauty of nature, there was no way I could ride a stationary bike. That would be too boring. I liked walking until I encountered coyotes on my walk two nights in a row. I've joined online exercise programs, and I do okay with these until I hurt my back. I can hurt my back sneezing. I need to exercise to strengthen my back. But it hurts, I tell myself, so I don't want to do more damage. I could do more damage tying my shoes, but I don't stop doing that.

I have an excuse for everything. I keep wondering when I will take my overall health seriously. What will it take for me to make permanent changes? A heart attack? Stroke? Cancer? I will continue my struggles to eat healthier and increase my physical activity, but I hope you will realize the importance of these habits early in your life and stick with them for good. I can remember my parents getting on health kicks when I was young. I remember once my mother decided we couldn't eat bread anymore, and she replaced it with flour tortillas. I cannot tell you the looks and questions I got at school because of my odd lunch. But nothing ever lasted too long. As an adult, I am repeating my parents' habits. I see my daughter following directly in my footsteps. If you can start these habits before you are pregnant, continue them throughout your pregnancy, and stay committed to them once your child or children are born, think of the example you will be setting. I can't change my past; I can only move forward. You have the blessing of making a commitment to health at a young age and continually moving forward in a healthy manner.

Glossary of Terms

The definitions of these terms come from medicinenet.com's MedTerm Medical Dictionary

Adaptogen – unique group of herbal ingredients used to improve the health of adrenal system.

Adrenal cortical function – produces steroid hormones which regulate carbohydrate and fat metabolism and mineralocorticoid hormones which regulate salt and water balance.

Adrenal gland – small gland located on top of kidneys. Produces hormones that control heart rate, blood pressure, the ways the body uses food, levels of mineral such as sodium and potassium in the blood, and other functions particularly involved in stress reactions.

Amenorrhea – absence of menstruation. Primary amenorrhea means period failed to occur during puberty. Secondary amenorrhea means menstruation started but stopped.

Amniocentesis – Before-birth diagnostic procedure in which a long needle is used to obtain amniotic fluid. This fluid can then be tested for genetic abnormalities in the developing fetus.

Analgesic – relieves pain.

Anemia – condition wherein a person has a lower-than-normal number of red blood cells or quantity of hemoglobin. Anemia diminishes the capacity of blood to carry oxygen.

Anovulation – absence of ovulation.

Antioxidants – a molecule that inhibits oxidation of other molecules. Oxidation reactions produce free radicals.

Antisperm antibodies–immunity to sperm. Can occur in women and men.

Astringent – causing the contraction of body tissues.

Anti-phospholipid antibody syndrome – immune system attacks normal proteins in body.

Autoimmune – misdirected immune response that occurs when the immune system begins to attack the body itself.

Autoimmune adrenal disease – condition wherein the adrenal glands do not produce hormones that can control blood pressure.

Autoimmune neuropathies – the body attacks the nervous system.

Autoimmune oophoritis/orchitis – inflammation of the ovary.

Autoimmune uveitis – inflammation of the eye. May be underlying cause of Behcet's disease.

Behcet's disease – inflammation of small blood vessels which can cause ulcers on genitalia.

Cervical mucus – nourishes and protects sperm on its journey to egg.

Chromosomal abnormalities – genetic abnormalities including but not limited to neural tube defect, congenital heart defect, cleft lip, limb defects, and urinary tract anomalies.

Crytorchidias – failure of one or both testicles to drop from the abdomen to the scrotum.

Cushing syndrome – excess of cortisol hormone.

Dehdroepiandrosterone – a steroid hormone made by adrenal gland and acts like testosterone and estrogen.

Down syndrome – common birth defect usually due to an extra chromosome. It causes mental retardation, characteristic facial appearances, and a multitude of other health issues and malformations.

Dysmenorrhea – painful periods

Electrolyte – substance that becomes ions that balance the electrolytes in our body necessary for normal function of cells and organs

Endocrine system – system in the body responsible for secreting hormones into bloodstream.

Endometriosis – presence of tissue that normally grows inside the uterus but is now found in abnormal anatomical location such as fallopian tubes (inside and out), ovaries, surface of uterus and intestines, and anywhere on surface of pelvic cavity.

Endometrium – inner layer of uterus

Enzymes – proteins that act as catalysts in mediating and speeding specific chemical reaction

Erectile dysfunction – consistent inability to sustain an erection sufficient for intercourse

Estradiol – primary female sex hormone and steroid.

Fibroids – common benign tumors of the uterus.

Follicle stimulating hormone – regulates the development, growth, pubertal maturation, and reproductive processes of the body.

Free radical – atoms or groups of atoms with an odd number of electrons. Free radicals seek out electrons to create matched pairs. They find matches in healthy cells, causing Injury to healthy cells, thus damaging DNA.

Gamma-linolenic acid – essential polyunsaturated fatty acid contained in evening primrose, borage oil, and black currant oil

Gene transcription – first step of gene expression. A particular segment of DNA is copied into RNA.

Grave's disease–over activity or toxicity of thyroid gland.

Guillain-Barre syndrome – progressive, systematic paralysis and loss of reflexes.

Hashimoto's thyroiditis – progressive disease of the thyroid gland. Antibodies attack the thyroid causing hypothyroidism.

Hirsutism – having excessive facial and body hair that can be a result of hormone imbalance

Hormones – chemical substance produced in the body that control the activity of certain organs and cells. Are essential for every activity of life, including digestion, metabolism, growth, reproduction, and mood control.

Hydrosalpinx – blocked fallopian tube that is filled with fluid.

Hypospadias – birth defect in which urethra opens on underside of penis.

Hysterosalpingogram – imaging test used to examine cavity of uterus and fallopian tubes.

Libido – sexual drive

Lignans – found in plants. Once ingested, they reduce risks of reproductive organ and colon cancer. They also improve cardiovascular health.

Linoleic acid – polyunsaturated omega-6 fatty acid.

Luteal Phase Defect – abnormality in endometrial develpment

Luteinizing hormone – hormone that affects sex organs. It's released from pituitary gland.

Lymphatic system – tissues and organs, including bone marrow, spleen, thymus, and lymph nodes, that produce and store cells that fight infection and disease.

Macrophage – type of white blood cells that ingests foreign material such as infectious microorganisms.

Menorrhagia – excessive menstrual bleeding

Metabolic waste – substances left over from excretory processes which may have lethal effects of not excreted.

Monocyte single-celled white blood cell able to ingest foreign material

Motility – ability of sperm to move properly through female reproductive tract or water to reach egg.

Mucus membrane – moist epithelial tissue that comes into contact with air.

Multiple sclerosis – disease in which there is a loss of myelin which coats the nerve fibers. Myelin serves as insulation and permits efficient nerve fiber conduction.

Myasthenia gravis – an autoimmune neuromuscular disease wherein the body mistakenly attacks its nicotinic acetylcholine receptors. These receptors transmit signals from the nervous system to the muscles.

Neural tube defect – major birth defect caused by abnormal development of neural tube. The neural tube is the structure present during embryonic life and gives rise to the central nervous system.

Oligomenorrhea – infrequent or light menstrual periods.

Ovarian cysts – a fluid-filled sac in ovary

Ovulation – release of ripe egg from ovary. Egg is released from surrounding cavity by a response to a hormone signal. Egg travels to fallopian tube and awaits fertilization.

Pelvic congestion – a congestion of blood in dilated veins of the pelvis. The ovarian vein and internal iliac vein can also be affected.

Pelvic inflammatory disease – ascending infection of female upper genital tract (Female structures above cervix). Most commonly caused by sexually transmitted diseases.

Photoestrogens – plant-derived xenoestrogens.

Pituitary gland – main endocrine gland. Produces hormones that control other glands and bodily functions.

Polycystic Ovarian Syndrome – irregular or no menstrual period.

Premature ovarian failure – loss of normal ovarian function before age 40.

Premenstrual Syndrome – combination of physical and mood disturbances occurring during last half of menstrual cycle. Normally ends with inset of menstrual flow.

Progesterone – principal female hormone that prepares the uterus to receive and sustain fertilized egg.

Prostaglandin – one of a number of hormone-like substances that participate in bodily functions like contration and relaxation of smooth muscle, dilation and constriction of blood vessels, control of blood pressure, and modulation of inflammation.

Recurrent miscarriage – frequently occurring miscarriages.

Salpingitis – infection and inflammation of fallopian tubes.

Stagnation – loss of blood flow to reproductive organs.

Temporal arteritis – inflammation of the walls of the blood vessels.

Testosterone – called a "male hormone." Sex hormone produced by testes that encourages development of male sexual characteristics, stimulates activity of male secondary sex characteristics, and prevents changes in them following castration.

Thyroid gland – makes and stores hormones that regulate heart rate, blood pressure, body temperature, and rate food is converted to energy.

T lymphocyte – white blood cell that protect the body from infection.

Type 1/immune medicated diabetes mellitus – the autoimmune system destroys pancreatic beta-cell. Results in failure to secrete insulin

Uterine adhesions – scar tissue build-up on interior wall of uterus.

Uterine hyperplasia – thickening of the lining of the uterus.

Wegener's granulumatosis – inflammation of small arteries and veins that supply blood to the tissues of the lungs, nasal passages, and kidneys.

Xenohormones – Cause progesterone deficiency in men and women.

Bibliography

"Antiphospholipid Syndrome." *mayoclinic.org.* 2015.

Barton-Schuster, Darlene, CH, "How to Use Herbs to Enhance Your Fertility Naturally," *natural-fertility-info.com.* 2014.

Berkley, Mike Dr. "Infertility and Chiropractic Care." *americanpregnancy.org.* February 2012.

Bouchez, Colette. "The Ancient Art of Infertility Treatment." *webmd.com.* October 13, 2003.

Boyd, Lucy J. "Foods and Fruits to Eat When You are Pregnant." *livestrong.com.* October 7, 2010.

Cohen, Juliet. "Natural Neuropathy Relief." *Autoimmune Neuropathy – Information, Treatment, and Prevention.*

Cram, Catherine. "Great Pregnancy Exercise." *babycenter.com.*

"Cushing Syndrome: Other FAQs." *nicd.nih.gov.* November 30, 2012.

"Diabetes Mellitus/Male Infertility." *ncbi.nlm.nih.gov.* 1990.

"Diseases and Conditions: Behcet"s Disease." *mayoclinic.org.* March 8, 2013.

"Diseases and Conditions: Female Infertility." *mayoclinic.org.* July 16, 2013.

"Diseases and Conditions: Vasculitis." *mayoclinic.org.* October 8, 2014.

"Diseases and Conditions: Wegener's Granulomatosis." *mayoclinic. org.* December 19, 2012.

Eades, Lucy. "Infertility Causes, Diagnosis and Treatment." *conceiveeasy.com.* June 15, 2012.

"Exercise During Pregnancy." *webmd.com.* September 2, 2014.

"Find a Vitamin or Supplement." *webmd.com.* 2009.

Franklin, Liz. *The Organic Seasonal Cookbook: Cooking for a Greener World.* Bath U.K.: Parragon Books, 2007.

"Getting Pregnant in Your 40s." *babycentre.co.uk.* April 2013.

Granger, Alyssia. "Infertility Natural Treatments." *natural-fertility-info.com.* September 18, 2012.

"Guillain-Barre Syndrome: Treatments and Drugs." *mayoclinic.org.* July 3, 2014.

"Herbal Remedies for Guillain-Barre Syndrome." *findhomeremedy. com.* 2014.

Hollingsworth, Dorothy R. "Hyperthyroidism in Pregnancy." *Werner's Thyroid Edition.*

"Infertility in Men." *pennstatehershey.adam.com.* December 21, 2013.

"Infertility in Men. In-Depth Report." *nytimes.com.* 2008.

Ioachimescu, Adriana G. "Diseases of the Adrenal Gland." *clevelandclinicmeded.com.* 2015.

Kim, Helen. "Can Acupuncture Boost my Fertility?" *babycenter.com.* 2015.

"Later Age Pregnancies." *umm.edu.* University of Maryland Medical Center. December 9, 2012.

Livshits, Anna, Daniel s. Seideman. "Fertility Issues in Women with Diabetes." *Women's Health* 5 (6) (2009): 701-707.

"MedTerms Medical Dictionary A-Z List." *medicinenet.com.* 2015.

"Menstruation and Pregnancy in Women with Myasthenia Gravis." *mgawpa.org.* 2009.

Palmcrantz, Erica, and Irmela Lilja. *Raw Food: A Complete Guide for Every Meal of the Day.* New York: Skyhorse Publishing, 2010.

"Penis Trauma and Injury–Herbal Erection Treatment." *herballove. com.*

"Pregnancy and Reproductive Issues." *nationalmssociety.org.*

Redberg, Dr. Rita F. *Betty Crooker Cookbook for Women – The Complete Guide to Women's Health and Wellness at Every Stage of Life.* Hoboken, NJ: Wiley Publishing, 2007.

"Temporal Arteritis." *nlm.nih.gov.* February 6, 2013.

"Treatments for Oophoritis." *rightdiagnosis.com.* June 17, 2014.

Rodriguez, Hethir, CH, CMT. "The Natural Fertility Diet. How to Eat for Optimal Fertility." *natural-fetility-info.com.* April 2015.

Scott, Monica, RN. "Natural Fertiltiy Boosters." *conceiveeasy.com.* February 10, 2013.

Smyth, Briohny. "Beautiful Belly." *dailyburn.com.* 2015.

"Structural Causes of Infertility." *fertilitynj.com.* Reproductive Science Center, New Jersey. 2015.

"Tests and Procedures Acupuncture." *mayoclinic.org.* February 21, 2015.

"Things to Consider if you Have MG and are Thinking about Getting Pregnant." *myasthenia.org.* 2010.

Thompson, Moly. "Are Zucchini and Squash OK for Pregnant Women?" *livestrong.com.* February 4, 2014

"Top Ten Foods High in Vitamin A, Potassium, Calcium." *healthaliciousness.com.* 2015.

"Twenty Best Foods for Fiber." *health.com.* 2015.

"Types of Diabetes Mellitus." *webmd.com.* 2015.

"Understanding Acupuncture." *newsinhealth.nih.gov.* February 2011.

Walsh, Beth MA. "Risk Factors for Chromosomal Abnormalities." *cvs.com.* May 2014.

Watson, K. "Pregnancy and Mental Health." *womenneuroscience. stanford.edu.* 2015.

"What is Peripheral Neuropathy (PN)?" *foundationforpn.org.*

Williams, Cody, DC. "The Chiropractic Approach to Infertility." *icpa4kids.org.* 2005.

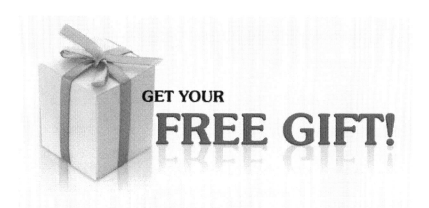

WAIT! – DO YOU LIKE FREE BOOKS?

My **FREE Gift** to You!! As a way to say **Thank You** for downloading

my book, I'd like to offer you more **FREE BOOKS!** Each time we

release a NEW book, we offer it first to a small number of people as

a test–drive. Because of your commitment here in downloading my

book, I'd love for you to be a part of this group. You can join easily

here ➔ **http://joylouisbooks.com/freebooks1**

CHECK OUT THESE #1 BEST SELLING

BOOKS FROM JOY LOUIS!

http://www.amazon.com/Joy-Louis/e/B00UMOZJE6

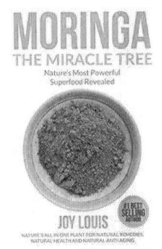
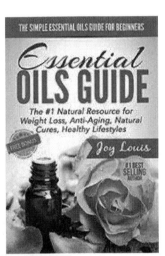

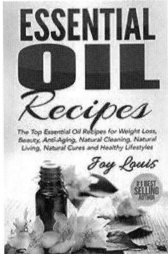

Conclusion

Thank you again for downloading this book!

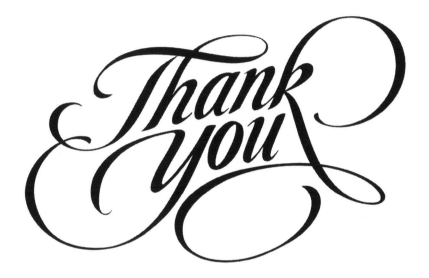

If you enjoyed this book, then I'd like to ask you for a favor, would you be kind enough to leave a review for this book on Amazon? It'd be greatly appreciated!

Help us better serve you by sending questions or comments to greatreadspublishing@gmail.com - Thank you!

29334162R00083

Made in the USA
Lexington, KY
29 January 2019